NURSE-PATIENT
COMMUNICATION

FOUNDATIONS OF NURSING SERIES

WM. C. BROWN COMPANY PUBLISHERS

ANNA KUBA
Consulting Editor

Nursing Observation
Virginia B. Byers
University of Pittsburgh

Nursing Observations of the Young Patient
Margaret A. Coffin
Boston University School of Nursing

Promotion of Physical Comfort and Safety
Valentina G. Fischer and Arlene F. Connolly
Boston University School of Nursing

Promoting Psychological Comfort
Gloria M. Francis and Barbara Munjas
Medical College of Virginia

Problem-Solving in Nursing Practice
Mae M. Johnson, Mary Lou C. Davis, and Mary Jo Bilitch

Nurse-Patient Communication
Garland K. Lewis
The Catholic University of America

Working with Others for Patient Care
Grace G. Peterson
DePaul University

The Teaching Function of the Nursing Practitioner
Margaret L. Pohl
Hunter College

Planning Patient Care
Lucile Lewis
Loma Linda University

Second Edition

NURSE-PATIENT COMMUNICATION

Garland K. Lewis
The Catholic University of America

WM. C. BROWN COMPANY PUBLISHERS, *Dubuque, Iowa*

Contents

Preface

Most people believe they communicate quite effectively—nurses are no exception. We in nursing are only beginning to recognize communication as an integral part of nursing care and have just begun to scratch the surface of this very complex function. Whenever human beings interact, they communicate, and we must recognize that communication is a highly important and necessary factor in all human endeavors.

This book is an introduction to the study of communication and is written as a resource on communication. The primary purpose is to alert all nurses to the significance of communication in all facets of nursing. Communication is the process whereby we give nursing care, or teach others to do so, or relate to nursing personnel or other professionals. Many references on various aspects of communication are provided in detail for the reader to examine. A second purpose, equally important, is that communication is a two-way process. The other person's perceptions are as valid as our own perceptions. To understand and communicate with another is to respect his perception.

Particular emphasis has been given to nonverbal communication and is presented within the framework of the senses. Additional information has been provided in this revision as there has been an increasing amount of interest from various disciplines on the importance of nonverbal aspects of communication. This study is important to all nurses in any setting in which they provide health care.

Communication has been described in breadth and in relation to certain specifics. Various technological developments are presented which have and will continue to influence our relations both nationally and internationally. The nurse will find the discussion of specific aspects of communication, namely, language, syntactics, interesting and useful in understanding how we derive meaning from our use of language. In addition, information from several theorists is presented relative to these aspects of verbal communication. Perceptions and feelings are discussed because they are basic to understanding communication.

Though this book is not designed as "how-to" communicate, some examples are given for clarification of the ideas presented. Specific attention is given to several components of nurse-patient communication and two additional components have been added in this revision. These were included because they were stimulated by student requests and questions about these two components. The five criteria for the examination of nurse-patient communication have been maintained. Woven throughout the book is a basic respect for man, which is a necessity if nurses are to learn to communicate effectively and truly develop relationships with the patients they serve.

Information as to how people learn to communicate has not been included, nor has pathological communication been considered. The first, though interesting, is omitted because of the many uncertainties about how we learn. Pathological communication was omitted in order to emphasize the preferred or positive learning, as too often health professionals learn about sickness rather than health.

The author wishes to express thanks and appreciation to her students for their enthusiasm and assistance; also appreciation to Gail Hartnett for her patience, time, and effort in the typing of the revised manuscript.

Garland K. Lewis

Communication

THE SCOPE OF COMMUNICATION

Communication! How often have you used that word lately? Man's fantastic ability to communicate with his fellowman is receiving more attention and study now than ever before in history. The whole of American society is attuned to the fact that communication is a highly important and necessary factor in all human endeavors. Ever since the early 1920s, when Benjamin Lee Wharf grasped the relationship between human language and human thinking, concern with communication has grown at a constantly accelerating rate.

Communication is now firmly implanted in the University curriculum, but is still generally considered to be interdisciplinary in nature. Mathematicians, sociologists, psychologists, philosophers, and anthropologists are all engaged in the study of communication. However, since communication is not yet considered to be a totally distinct discipline in most Universities, students must cross over various disciplines to obtain the variety of courses available. The past few years have seen opportunities opening up for the study of communication on the graduate level, and some doctoral dissertations have been done in this area.

In the field of medicine, a few neurophysiologists but mainly psychiatrists, have evidenced an interest in communication. Because psychotherapy is dependent on the patients' communication, both verbal and nonverbal communication has become a primary focus of the psychiatrist's study. Nursing has only recently begun to recognize the importance of communication in nurse-patient relationships. It is a rarity to find the subject a part of the nursing curriculum. It is my belief that we have long neglected communication as a necessary component within the curriculum, particularly as it relates to the nurse-patient interactions. The scientific knowledge we possess regarding the broad spectrum of health and illness is of little value if we are unable to interact with our patients. The basis of all our interactions rests on our ability to communicate with our patients. It is my belief that many of our dilemmas in nursing stem from our inability to understand our patients and to recognize our responsibility in the communication process. From many of the studies related to patients' assessment of their care, it becomes apparent that the failures in communication have been a prime source of distress. We have a moral obligation to learn how to communicate effectively.

Communication is a central part of everything we do in life. The way we dress communicates information about our age, economic status, and frequently our profession or occupation. Our behavior and speech communicate much about our education, our location of birth, our feelings toward others and our moods. The newspapers and magazines we read, our church affiliation, our choice of clubs, restaurants, automobiles, and the structure and location of our homes, all communicate information about the kind of person we are and the values we hold. It is through this kind of communication that we convey information about ourselves to others.

Communication involves more than verbal, explicit, or intentional messages. It includes all the processes by which people influence one another. All actions, incidents, or happenings function communicatively. Each encounter that we have with other individuals provides us with additional information about them, and influences our perception of them. All human interactions succeed or fail because of our communication with each other. Whether the interaction is between two individuals or a group, whether it takes place in a school, a hospital, a business, a state department or between nations, the basic ingredient is communication.

One way that communication helps or hinders relationships between people can be seen in the United States foreign aid program. Many critics of the program state that although the United States has spent hundreds of millions of dollars in helping less fortunate nations, it does not enjoy the esteem or affection of these countries. Part of the reason for this could very well lie in the fact that we, as a nation, do not understand foreign cultures well enough to be able to communicate effectively with them. The misunderstandings that result from this basic lack of communication have caused other nations to be suspicious and even resentful toward us.

It is perhaps being an apostle of the obvious to point out that culture and communication are inextricably related. A. G. Smith reinforces this idea by stating that, "In modern society different people communicate in different ways, as do people in different societies around the world;

and the way people communicate is the way they live. It is their culture. Who talks with whom? How? And about what."[1] It is necessary to make the relationship between culture and communication explicit in order to understand why the interest in the field has become so pervasive. Culture affects communication in various ways. It determines the time and timing of interpersonal events, the places where it is appropriate to discuss particular topics, the physical distance separating one speaker from another, and the tone of voice that is appropriate to the subject matter. Culture differences affect the relationship of what is said to what is meant—as when "no" means "maybe" and "tomorrow" means "never."

The scope of communication is so broad that only a brief orientation can be given of the total field. We should be aware, however, of the focus of current theoretical developments, and possess a knowledge of the variety of professions involved in the numerous investigations. Dr. Alfred Smith in his text, *Culture and Communication,* discusses the three major theories of human communication, and the three kinds of professional investigators involved in the development of these theories. The following is a brief resumé of his presentation.

The mathematical theory of communication has been developed by special kinds of mathematicians: electrical engineers, theoretical physicists, and communication analysts. These investigators are concerned with the technical transmission of messages by means of radio, television, or computers. They are also concerned with the specialized study known as cybernetics.[2] Norbert Wiener defines cybernetics as the "attempts to find the common elements in the functioning of automatic machines and of the human nervous system, and to develop a theory which will cover the entire field of control and communications in machines and in living organisms."[3] For a number of years, the Josiah Macy, Jr. Foundation has sponsored conferences on cybernetics, which brought physicians, engineers, and psychiatrists together to promote meaningful communication between scientific disciplines and to share the knowledge of these disciplines. Studies in medicine relate to automatic changes in our physiological systems which involve the feedback and transmitting of information.

The second major theory is the social-psychological theory developed by social psychologists. This group is mainly concerned with analyses of the interactions of groups of people. Some investigators focus on the social aspects of communication, and some focus on the psychological aspects.

---

[1] Alfred G. Smith, *Communication and Culture* (New York: Holt, Rinehart & Winston, Inc., 1966), p. 1.
[2] *Ibid.,* pp. 1-14.
[3] *Ibid.,* pp. 64-65.

The latter analyze human codes and networks which are analogous to the coding of the mathematical theorists. The former have concentrated on examining social cohesiveness, leadership, and other properties of face-to-face groups. Their analysis is based on the formal observation and analyses of specific kinds of interactions.

The third major theory—the linguistic theory—is the concern of linguistic anthropologists. Their primary focus is the analysis of the spoken languages of the various peoples of the world. The aim of these theorists is "to develop a model and a procedure for making a complete, concise, and objective description of the speech of a people: the phonology, the grammar, and the other parts of English and of all other languages."[4]

From this brief review, it becomes evident that the study of communication is quite comprehensive in subject material, method of study, and variety of disciplines. It should be noted that the framework for all of these studies is mathematical theory, based on empirical data. Other sociologists, psychologists, linguists, and particularly semanticists have been less rigid in their study of communication, but have added to the general knowledge of the field. In some instances they have questioned the mathematical models for examining the communication process. Some of their contributions will be included later on.

Although I have mentioned mass communication previously, I would like to make some specific comments on this phenomenon, since it wields such a great influence on our society. This system of communication is frequently controlled by people who have little interest in the influence of the message, apart from the monetary gain from the sale of their product. Radio, television, motion pictures, and the press are all mediums of mass selling to millions of consumers. Too often, the production of the program takes precedence over its consequences and impact. Marshall McLuhan has become the twentieth-century critic of the electronic mass media of our culture. He believes that "the medium is the message" in terms of the electronic age, and that a totally new environment has been created which has adversely influenced our thoughts, our senses, our actions, and in turn our communication with each other. He views all of these media as having a simultaneous impact on our senses, at a terrific speed, and with instant translation. Where previously we translated one kind of sensory experience to our other senses, and arrived at a unified image, today, many senses are bombarded at once, but the experience itself is missing.[5]

---

[4]*Ibid.*, pp. 119-120.
[5]Marshall McLuhan, *Understanding Media: The Extensions of Man* (New York: The New American Library, Inc., 1964), pp. 23-35.

For many years, we have been aware that mass communication can strongly affect the general population. It would seem that there is a very definite relationship between the glorification of guns in television commercials, television programs, and motion pictures, and the series of assassinations that have occurred during the 1960s. It is very difficult to offer scientific proof of this, however, since controlled psychological testing of the population is thus far an impossible task. We can advance some rather convincing theories about this relationship, however, based on the adverse effects that television news coverage had on the summer, 1967 violence in Detroit and Newark.

Dr. Hayakawa, a noted professor of semantics, says we need to discover ways of making more accurate assessment of the influence of mass communications, because at present we have no idea how all of these media affect the general population. We do not even know for sure how many minutes of an hour are devoted to commercials. We really don't know what the communication media is doing to us.[6]

What looms as an important concern of the next decade is international television. Intercultural communication is even more complex than communication within a given culture. We now have the Telstar, Syncom, and Early Bird satellite communication systems which link us with specific countries. Don R. Browne,[7] who has worked with the United States Office of Information, predicts that within the next decade it may be possible (barring several problems) for us to receive and send daily international programs. The four main problem areas he foresees are: (a) technical, (b) economic, (c) legal, and (d) sociopsychological. The sociopsychological and economic problems would seem to present the major barriers to be overcome before daily transmission can become a reality.

We live in a world in which the distance between continents shrinks daily, and the proximity of our fellowman in urban areas increases at an alarming rate. Our ability to live with each other at home and our relations with those abroad depends upon our ability to understand each other. Technologically, we are capable of producing much more than we are willing or able to handle sociologically. The Federal Communications Commission lacks many regulations for the licensing of current television productions, and new rules need to be established to handle emerging developments.

---

[6]S. I. Hayakawa, "Communications in the Coming Decade," *Proceedings of the 1967 Institute in Technical and Industrial Communications* (Colorado State University, September, 1967), pp. 1-11.

[7]Don R. Browne, "Problems in International Television," *Journal of Communication*, Vol. 17, September, 1967, pp. 198-209.

Many of the social ills of our country are related to our inadequate communication on the personal as well as governmental levels. The inherent threat from our inability to communicate effectively may be disastrous to our civilization, if we do not adequately solve this problem.

COMMUNICATION IN THE YEAR 2000

What can we anticipate for the future in the field of communication? Dr. Francis Cartier, research editor of the *Journal of Communication*, predicts there will be three-dimensional television and long distance telephone dialing available and in use all over the globe. Electric typewriters will be able to talk to one another, and we may have a machine which will type what is dictated to it.[8] The Bell Telephone Company will expand their Picturephone, see-while-you-talk service, which is already in limited use. By the year 2000, they may be able to provide this service in three dimensions and full color. The cordless, portable extension phone, which can be carried anywhere, is already being tested. The Bell Telephone Company predicts that you will be able to lock your door or turn down the thermostat by calling your house with your car telephone, and then simply touching a few buttons. For the housewife, the computer will provide a list of the supplies needed, the amount of each, and then order them from the stores offering the best bargains.[*]

Medically, it will be possible for your physician to obtain by computer an entire medical history for diagnosis. Sensors attached to your body could send a report of your symptoms to the doctor, with a summary of everything he will need to know about your particular problem. These possibilities are a direct result of the interdisciplinary activity of biomedical engineering. Engineers are helping to devise artificial limbs, as well as precise instruments for surgery. The mechanical engineer assists with air pollution analysis; the aeronautical engineer examines the physiological effects of space travel on man; and the electrical engineer has devised the heart-pacing machine.

Does all of this within the next sixty years seem difficult to believe? Television, satellites, computers, and even telephones were impossible dreams only a hundred years ago. Scientists will be able to accomplish all of this, and probably more. What they can't foresee is whether people will want to make use of these innovations in their daily lives, or whether they will prefer to put them to other uses.

---

[8]Francis A. Cartier, "The Study of Communications in 1970," *Journal of Communication*, Vol. 10, March, 1960, p. 196.
[*]Taken from "The C & P Call," Vol. 39, May, 1968.

Computers will soon become, directly or indirectly, an integral part of the daily life of the majority of people. Leighton C. Wood looks at how some computers and their communications are being used, and reminds us that the commercial computer business is only fifteen years old. The Federal Bureau of Investigation plans to create a nationwide computer network. Fifteen states are already tied in with the National Center in Washington. Real estate associations are developing telephone terminals linked to computers. Detroit now has such a system with 4,000 homes listed. Within seconds, the computer can scan all listings which fit a prospective buyer's requirements. Electrocardiograms will soon be done in the patient's room or at home. The results will be telephoned to the computer, which will analyze signals and provide the physician with a fast reading. The Federal Aviation Agency plans to use computers for nationwide automatic control of air traffic, from take-off to landing. The system has already been installed at Atlantic City and Jacksonville, Florida. International Business Machines has a nationwide internal communications network, controlled from a computing center at their headquarters, which enables them to transmit messages among their major offices, plants, and laboratories throughout Canada, Europe, Japan, and the United States. Some 24,000 messages are transmitted each day, and they anticipate that these will double in two years.[9]

These are only some samples; there are many more. We must recognize that change is occurring rapidly, and that the pace will be accelerated. A crucial question is—are we as individuals ready for these changes? The need for continued education becomes paramount if we are to deal with these rapidly changing and complex communication problems.

Thorrel B. Fest is concerned about the overwhelming mass of information we are collecting, and asks, "how can the responsible individual at any level cope with what he should know in order to function fully and effectively?" He further questions the kind of system we need for the management and control of this flood of information. If electronic equipment can provide our medical history and our credit rating at the press of a button, how will we use this technology productively and constructively?

Another crucial question results from this accumulation of personal data—how do we maintain respect for privacy, integrity, and security of information regarding the individual person? In addition, if we provide internationally televised programs, what kind of information will we feed to the underdeveloped nations? We are already concerned with the kind

---

[9]Leighton C. Wood, "Computers and Communications," *Proceedings of the 1967 Institute in Technical and Industrial Communications* (Colorado State University, September, 1967), pp. 126-131.

of information available to the delinquent, disturbed, suicide-prone, and socially angry individuals within our society.[10] We have only begun to think of the possibilities from these new dimensions. As yet we do not know, nor have we adequately considered, the consequences of our technological discoveries.

Dr. Cartier believes that though we have made vast progress in these miracle machines, we will not be any nearer to understanding the processes of human communication. He indicates that we will probably know more, but that we won't understand that much more, because the more knowledgeable we become, the more complex our problems become.[11]

DEFINITION OF COMMUNICATION

Various experts have defined communication, and disagreement exists among them. In fact, there is no generally accepted definition. In 1960, John B. Newman noted that "communication" is not even restricted to process. It also encompasses a body of knowledge and a field of study, including listening. He enumerates the many problems involved in delineating a definition, and suggests a rationale for a pragmatic one. Such a definition would "seek *a* meaning *for* Communication," which would permit all persons concerned with communication to speak intelligibly to one another.[12] We are prone to want a definition for the words we use, even though we frequently do not adhere to the preciseness of the dictionary. Dr. Newman also notes that a definition in a dictionary records past practices in using a word, and is thus a form of history, and not a statement of unchangeable fact.

But for our purposes here, we are mainly concerned with interpersonal communication. That is, communication which occurs between a nurse and a patient. For this reason it is necessary to define communication as a process; it is continuous and involves many changes. Our perceptions of ourselves and our perceptions of the other person must be included as well as our verbal and nonverbal messages. Communication with another includes all the processes by which people influence one another. This includes all aspects of our culture. Simply stated, interpersonal communication is the attempt to understand the other person's point of view,

---

[10]Thorrel B. Fest, "Significant Issues in Communication: Identification and Resolution," *Proceedings of the 1967 Institute in Technical and Industrial Communications* (Colorado State University, September, 1967), pp. 126-131.

[11]Cartier, *op. cit.*, p. 10.

[12]John B. Newman, "A Rationale for a Definition of Communication," *Communication and Culture*, A. G. Smith, (ed.) (New York: Holt, Rinehart & Winston, Inc., 1966), pp. 55-63.

from his frame of reference, which includes his feelings about the situation.

We need to be cognizant that we communicate every time an idea or thought is conveyed to and understood by another person. If I do not understand what you are saying—or your words do not have meaning for me—we are not communicating. It is not necessary that I agree with what you are saying. As long as I understand you, communication has taken place.

PURPOSE OF COMMUNICATION

More important than a definition of communication, however, is the aim or function of communication. A review of a variety of authors' comments on purpose or aim reveals differences and similarities of beliefs. All seem to agree that communication involves the transmission of messages from one person to another, but not all agree that this is the major purpose. Some experts place their emphasis on the verbal content of the message. That is, they see language as the code of human interaction. In a sentence, each word is related to other words, according to their position within the sentence. This is known as syntactics. Meaning depends on the structure of the words.

The aim of communication as seen by another group is the transfer of ideas from one person to another. A person learns through his culture. His language, gestures, spacial and temporal relations, all have meaning. Language is a part of behavior. What is described is semantics—the study of human interaction through the mechanisms of linguistic communication. This should not be confused with the original meaning of semantics, which was the historical study of the changes in the meaning of words.

David Berlo and Dean Barnlund agree that both of these aims are constituent elements of communication, but feel that neither comprise the entire purpose of communication. They see the purpose as a process of creating a meaning. The meanings are *not* in the message, but in the message-user. Berlo says that the purpose is "the goal of a creator or receiver of a message rather than the property of the message itself."[13] More broadly, he says "we attempt to become an affecting agent, to affect others, our physical environment and ourselves."

Both of these authors focus on the person more than on the words in the message. They regard the state of mind, the assumptive world, and the needs of the listener as primarily important in communication. Barn-

---

[13]David K. Berlo, *The Process of Communication* (New York: Holt, Rinehart & Winston, Inc., 1960), p. 10.

lund says that the "aim of communication is to increase the number and consistency of our meanings within the limits set by patterns of evaluation that have proven successful in the past, our emerging needs and drives, and the demands of the physical and social setting of the moment."[14] We communicate because we need to reduce uncertainty, to act effectively, and to defend or strengthen the ego.

Berlo is even more specific regarding meaning—"meanings are in people," they are learned and are our own personal property. We learn meanings, we add to them, we distort them, forget them, change them. They are in us, not in the messages. Thus our aim is "to communicate and to influence—to affect with intent."[15]

When we speak of "meaning" we are getting into less known territory. Meanings are more complex and less objective. There has been less study done in this area than in the transmission of messages or the content of messages. Barnlund makes the point that meanings are generated from within the person—messages are generated from the outside.

From the discussion of the purpose of communication, we find discrepancies in the views of various theorists. It is not our purpose to decide the merits of the theories, but to realize that all three approaches contribute to our understanding of why we communicate. The choice of emphasis marks the distinction between each approach.

SUCCESSFUL COMMUNICATION

How do we know when we have successfully communicated with another person? Are you certain that your patient understands you? What criteria have you developed for assurance that he has received your message? To communicate effectively, you must first of all recognize that different words mean different things to different people. For example, the word hostile does not mean the same to all people. Your use of it may be to describe what I would consider angry or annoyed. Words have little intrinsic meaning. A great part of their meaning is determined by the context in which they appear.

Another criteria for effective communication is the way in which we organize our messages: how we describe our experiences, how we classify events, what style we use, how correctly we use grammar, or how elaborate our words are. Consider the following sentence taken from a letter to a county welfare department. "I'm glad to report my husband who was reported missing is dead." The humor of this statement is caused

---

[14]Dean C. Barnlund, "Toward a Meaning-Centered Philosophy of Communication," *ETC: A Review of General Semantics,* Vol. 20, December, 1963, p. 458.
[15]Berlo, *op. cit.,* p. 12.

by the fact that it is inadequately structured and does not convey the intended meaning. On the other hand, contrast the difference between the humor caused by the structure of the above quotation with the following: "What is purple and hums?" Answer, "An electric grape." "Why does it hum?" Answer, "Because it doesn't know the words."[16] Humor is present in both, and the words of both are correct. In the first example the humor derives from the faulty structure. In the second, the humor derives from the juxtaposition of unusual ideas. In this second example, personal experience, level of abstraction, and individual perception are all constituent factors in the recognition of the humor. These three factors are also important to the effectiveness of our communication.

Earlier, it was mentioned that the aim of communication was to influence or affect another person. If this is so, successful communication would then depend on whether the meaning conveyed leads to the desired conduct of the receiver of the message. This requires knowing how you intend to affect the other person. Berlo exemplifies this point when he notes that teachers forget about the influence they want to exert on students when they "concentrate on covering the material" or "filling fifty minutes three times a week."[17]

Communication is effective when rational judgments are facilitated. This applies both to individuals or groups. Rational judgments can be arrived at when meanings are shared and there is respect for each other's ideas. Communication is more accurate when there is free feedback between persons. When an individual feels free to ask questions, he arrives at a better understanding of what another is trying to communicate. There is more certainty and confidence developed if feedback is adequate. Communication is also more effective when nonverbal messages are recognized, acknowledged, and accurately interpreted. Communication that is nonthreatening aids the flow of information and conveys a sincere interest toward others, facilitating positive interactions. The real value of effective communication lies in its ability to increase understanding among men.

BIBLIOGRAPHY

BARNLUND, DEAN C. "Toward a Meaning-Centered Philosophy of Communication," *ETC: A Review of General Semantics*, December, 1963.

BERLO, DAVID K. *The Process of Communication*. New York: Holt, Rinehart & Winston, Inc., 1960.

BROWNE, DON R. "Problems in International Television," *Journal of Communication*, September, 1967.

---

[16]McLuhan, *op. cit.*, p. vii.
[17]Berlo, *op. cit.*, p. 13.

CARTIER, FRANCIS A. "The Study of Communications in 1970," *Journal of Communication*, March, 1960.

FEST, THORREL B. "Significant Issues in Communication: Identification and Resolution," *Proceedings of the 1967 Institute in Technical and Industrial Communications*, Colorado State University, September, 1967.

HAYAKAWA, S. I. "Communications in the Coming Decade," *Proceedings of the 1967 Institute in Technical and Industrial Communications*, Colorado State University, September, 1967.

McLUHAN, MARSHALL. *Understanding Media: The Extensions of Man.* New York: The New American Library, Inc., 1964.

NEWMAN, JOHN B. "A Rationale for a Definition of Communication," *Communication and Culture*, A. G. Smith, (ed.). New York: Holt, Rinehart & Winston, Inc., 1966.

SMITH, ALFRED G. *Communication and Culture* (ed.). New York: Holt, Rinehart & Winston, Inc., 1966.

WOOD, LEIGHTON C. "Computers and Communications," *Proceedings of the 1967 Institute in Technical and Industrial Communications*, Colorado State University, September, 1967.

Language

LANGUAGE AS SYMBOLS

The ability to talk is man's greatest human achievement. Even the most primitive human cultures have their complete and grammatical language. No tribe has ever been found without a well-developed language.

Edward Sapir, an anthropologist whose work centered mainly on American Indian languages and cultures, states that "language is primarily a system of phonetic symbols for the expression of communicable thought and feeling."[1] There is no question that language is symbolic, and that man's distinctive ability is that he has learned to use symbols. Other authors also note this feature. Harry Warfel notes that this concept of symbolism is applicable not only to the English language, but also to every one of the other three thousand or so identified tongues:

> Language is a structured system of overt, learned and therefore non-instinctive, sequentially produced, voluntary, human, symbol-carrying vocal sounds by which communication is carried on between two or more persons.[2]

Sapir makes the point that language is not instinctive in nature, but is learned. Susanne Langer, a philosopher, agrees with this. "Language . . . is none the less a product of sheer learning, an art handed down from generation to generation, and where there is no teacher there is no accomplishment." She describes language in the following way. "In language we have the free, accomplished use of symbolism, the record

---

[1]Edward Sapir, *Culture, Language and Personality* (Los Angeles: University of California Press, 1960), p. 1.
[2]Harry R. Warfel, *Language a Science of Human Behavior* (Cleveland: Howard Allen, Inc., 1962), p. 29.

of articulate conceptual thinking; without language there seems to be nothing like explicit thought whatever."[3] She goes a step further when she indicates that without language we are without explicit thought. In other words, our language is the tool by which we organize our thinking into meaningful symbols.

What are symbols, and what do they stand for? Langer describes symbols as "vehicles for the conception of objects." She clarifies this further in the following statement. "In talking about things we have conceptions of them, not the things themselves; and it *is the conceptions, not the things,* that symbols directly mean. Behavior toward conceptions is what words normally evoke; this is the typical process of thinking."[4]

We must understand that the word is a symbol of a thing, not the thing itself; it stands for or symbolizes our conception of the thing named. As an illustration, let us consider the word "bamboo." To most persons, it is a symbol for a particular plant. To persons who have seen the plant, and have also seen furniture made from bamboo, there would be an additional dimension to the conception symbolized by the word. To others, the word may symbolize a fishing pole, a food, or a whistle. On the other hand, to some people, the word might not symbolize anything. A child in Alaska might learn the word from the dictionary, but have no conception of it other than it being a plant. Likewise a child in Florida could learn that the word "igloo" meant a type of dwelling, but it would have little meaning for him as a dwelling. Thus, it is not the "thing" (in this case, the igloo or bamboo) that the word denotes, but the connotations or the meaning conveyed by the symbol. It becomes obvious that the more we learn about a particular thing, the more our conception of it increases. Words can also be signs, according to Langer, but "signs indicate the existence—past, present, or future—of a thing, event, or condition." Wet streets are a sign that it has rained, a smell of smoke is a sign of existing fire, and dawn is a sign of the impending sunrise. There is a difference, however, between the function of a sign or a symbol. Langer makes this following distinction: signs announce their objects to the person, whereas symbols lead the person to conceive their objects.[5]

The primary function of signs and *symbols in language* is to facilitate communication. Our knowledge of reality is determined by the way that we conceive it verbally, and the way that our experiences are transformed into concepts which can be verbally expressed. In Chapter 1, it

---

[3]Susanne K. Langer, *Philosophy in a New Key* (New York: The New American Library, Inc., 1951), pp. 94-98.

[4]*Ibid.*, p. 61.

[5]*Ibid.*, p. 58.

was noted that communication and culture are inseparable. We can see how our culture is expressed through language.

Hayakawa adds the dimension of semantics to his definition of language in the following statement: "A language is therefore not merely the system of signs but also the whole repertory of semantic reactions which the signs produce in those who speak and understand the language. The structural assumptions implicit in a language are of necessity reflected in behavior reactions."[6]

Aldous Huxley indicates the value of language to society in the following statement:

> . . . for language makes it possible for men to build up the social heritage of accumulated skill, knowledge and wisdom, thanks to which it is possible for us to profit by the experience of past generations, as though they were our own. . . . The existence of language permits human beings to behave with a degree of purposefulness, perseverance and consistency unknown among the other mammals and comparable only to the purposefulness, perseverance and consistency of insects acting under the compulsive force of instinct.[7]

Language is our means of social interaction, and Hayakawa believes that "cooperation through the use of language is the fundamental mechanism of human survival."[8] The way in which language is used can also result in disagreements, argument, and conflict. When conflict occurs, it is usually because both parties are not communicating; one is not understanding the words of another. Thus, language can be used to promote cooperation or to create conflict. Harry Warfel emphasizes this point in relation to the young in our society:

> . . . language is the instrument by which youth makes its peace with, or gets into trouble, in society. Only with language can youth open doors into areas of new knowledge. Only with language can youth put itself on a fair road to a full, reasoned, knowledgeable understanding of an adult's duties, opportunities, and responsibilities.[9]

Harry Hoijer, a noted researcher in linguistics, informs us that the first written records in English appear about A.D. 900 and "examination of the records reveals that from A.D. 900 to the present, a period of little more than 1000 years, English has changed radically in pronunciation,

---

[6]S. I. Hayakawa, *Language, Meaning and Maturity* (New York: Harper & Row, Publishers, 1954), p. 218.

[7]Aldous Huxley, *Words and Their Meanings* (Los Angeles: The Ward Ritchie Press, 1940), p. 13.

[8]S. I. Hayakawa, *Language in Thought and Action* (New York: Harcourt, Brace & World, Inc., 1949), p. 22.

[9]Warfel, *op. cit.*, p. 179.

grammar, and vocabulary."[10] This information is of interest not only in regard to the antiquity of our language but also to our modern language. Our modern language is characterized by a rapidly expanding vocabulary from the arts, sciences, and professions, giving evidence of new ideas and new knowledge. As new ideas emerge, we require new words to express them. Compare a textbook on nursing or medicine published in the 1800s with a current publication, and notice the differences in vocabulary.

LINGUISTICS

As previously mentioned, the study of a language, particularly our spoken language, is called linguistics. The structural units of a language are phonemes (sound units) and morphemes (grammatical units). Morphemes are words or parts of words that are arranged systematically according to the grammar of our language. Patterns of sounds combine into words, and words become elements of a sentence having a relationship to each other. This relationship of part to part is called syntax. Linguistic descriptions emphasize patterns and structures of a language.

Dr. E. A. Hoebel, an anthropologist, makes an interesting comment regarding the rules of grammar: "Although firm grammatical rules control the use of every language, the rules are not made by grammarians. They have been naively arrived at by generations of speakers who had no consciousness of what they were doing."[11] I'm sure that many pupils have attributed the rules of grammar to their teachers.

The development of our American language has been influenced by various sociological, historical, geographical, and ethnological conditions. Colloquial speech has altered with rapidly changing patterns of American life.

One interesting phenomenon in the development of our language has been the adoption of a certain word within a particular section of our country that has not been accepted in another. The word "prairie," for instance, is used in one section of the country, and "meadow" in another, though both refer to grassland. We use the term *dialect* to explain these regional differences of words.

In many instances, words are pronounced differently in various sections of a country. The word "tennis" is pronounced "tinnis" in the Mid-

---

[10]Harry Hoijer, "Language in Culture," Patrick and Mary Hazard (eds.), *Language and Literacy To-Day* (Chicago: Science Research Associates, Inc., 1965), p. 34.

[11]E. Adamson Hoebel, *Man in the Primitive World* (2d ed.) (New York: McGraw-Hill Book Co., 1958), p. 561.

west. In the United States, as in England, we all speak the English language, but we speak and use certain words that are different in specific sections of the country. Dr. Hans Kurath, a retired professor of English, has spent many years examining the dialects of the United States. He has compiled a linguistic Atlas of New England as a first step toward a survey of all the United States and Canada. From the work of Professor Kurath we can see that within the broad area divisions of the North, South, and Central United States, there are further subdivisions of local dialects within these broad geographical areas. He has found, for example, a significant number of differences between the speech of people in Michigan and Wisconsin.*

SEMANTICS

Semantics can be defined as the science of meaning. Dr. S. I. Hayakawa, an anthropologist, has contributed significantly to the field of semantics, and has, through a variety of activities, brought the relevance of general semantics to millions of people both in the United States and abroad. He states that semantics may be defined in three ways: (1) the study of laws and conditions under which signs and symbols, including words, may be meaningful; (2) the study of the relationship between language, thought, and behavior, that is, how human action is influenced by words, whether spoken by others or to oneself in thought; (3) the historical study of changes in the meaning of words.[12] Meaning is partially dependent on structure (phonemes and morphemes), but there is also the assigned meaning, which refers to denotative and connotative meaning.

Linguistics and semantics are closely related, but semantics is more concerned with the way in which people communicate with each other. Interest in semantics in the United States began in the 1930s, and was largely influenced by Alfred Korzybski, a Polish-American scholar and engineer. His main thesis is that language is not only a necessary tool for thought and communication, but also a whole body of assumptions about ourselves and the world, which in part determines the kinds of thoughts we are able to have.

Stuart Larick in *ETC: A Review of General Semantics*,[13] reviews Korzybski's major works and explains the need of general semantics. Korzyb-

---

*For a more specific breakdown, see Patrick D. and Mary E. Hazard, *Language and Literacy Today*, "Regional Variations" by Albert H. Marckwardt, pp. 93-103.
[12]Hayakawa, *Language, Meaning and Maturity*, op. cit., p. 119.
[13]Stuart Larick, "Why 'General' Semantics?," *ETC: A Review of General Semantics*, Vol. 29, No. 2, June, 1972, pp. 181-185.

ski believed that man could learn how to think and communicate more successfully in his everyday life if he learned how to reason more logically. He believed that we should use the methods of the scientist, which is to revise premises when they no longer fit the facts, and correct previous evaluations. People who cling to rigid formulas of behavior do not learn to revise generalizations or "laws" and become static.

Larick discusses how we use symbols—for example, a symbol that stands for a tree.

> We can manipulate this symbol, we can visualize it as taller or greener, or covered with snow. When we wish to convey information about the tree to another person, we don't pick up the object and place it inside him. What we transmit are symbols, the most common of which are spoken or written words. But the word "tree" is not in itself a tree; an actual tree is a living thing, changing from year to year, season to season, even instant to instant. *The symbol that stands for it can never express all its infinite characteristics.* A human being can only abstract some of its features, and no two people will ever select all the same elements.[14]

Larick states that "Korzybski was convinced that symbols govern our behavior: we feel, think, and act according to what we build up inside ourselves." Also, "that if we could respond more sanely to symbols we would have a vital key to emotional maturity and mental health." A broader view though, would go beyond semantics and encompass "the entire process of observing (or sensing) an event, structuring the internal image of it, and responding to it." It was to this process that Korzybski applied the term, General Semantics. During the past thirty-five years, many other specialists and scholars from a variety of disciplines have studied meaning in relation to language and symbolism. A tremendous amount of investigation has been done regarding the relationship between language and meaning and the effect that our use of words has on others. According to A. G. Smith, the only group of specialists not interested in semantics or the meaning of messages are the mathematicians, who feel that cultural processes are beyond the scope of mathematical theory.[15]

A great deal of controversy surrounds the term "meaning." Some people believe that meaning is conveyed by words, or the sequence of words —their structure; others believe that meaning is to be found in the reactions to the words, and still others contend that the meanings are in the individual, not in the messages transmitted. The latter insist that

---

[14]*Ibid.*, p. 183.
[15]Alfred G. Smith, *Communication and Culture* (New York: Holt, Rinehart & Winston, Inc., 1966), p. 6.

when we learn meanings, they become a part of us. We communicate when and if we find others who hold similar meanings. There is, of course, some uniformity of meaning within words, or we would not be able to communicate at all.

Basic to our understanding of meaning is the knowledge of the difference between denotative and connotative meanings of words. Denotative meaning refers to word-object relationships. It is a relationship that exists between the object in the physical world and the word that stands for that object. The words "horse," "chairs," etc., are examples of things in our physical world. Of course, we must realize that these are only approximations. Not all horses are alike, nor are all chairs alike. If the object is visible, you can point to it and say, "This is a horse," and others will know exactly what is meant. If the horse were not present, you might say "My horse won the race." In this case, however, further explanation would be needed about the kind of horse and the kind of race, etc. This explanation leads us to connotative meanings of words. Connotative meaning is person-oriented. It is a relationship between the object and the person, and is usually related to a personal experience. In other words, it is our description of an object as we perceive it.

Connotative meanings can easily lead to misunderstandings because they are somewhat different for each of us. Consider the word "freedom" or the phrase "black power." Both of these terms have highly personal connotative meanings. This is why it is often difficult to discuss or arrive at a consensus about the meaning of "freedom" or "black power."

Semantic meaning includes both the denotative and connotative functions of words. To understand the precise meaning of any sentence, we must consider the total context, including the way that the sentence relates to other sentences, as well as the whole background relevant to the message. Many misunderstandings can occur because we have taken a sentence or a word out of the context of the total message. To make sense, each expression contributes to the whole, of which it is a part.

We use our language to express and elicit meanings. Because meanings are personal, they differ from person to person, and because meaning is the substance of language, we can see why communication is so complex. Within our highly competitive society, the ability to communicate is imperative, if we are to become effective citizens. John Gardner's remarks are highly significant:

> A complex society is dependent every hour of every day upon the capacity of its people to read and write, to make complex judgments and to act in the light of fairly extensive information.[16]

---

[16]John W. Gardner, *Excellence* (New York: Harper & Row, Publishers, 1961), p. 35.

Even from this brief review of language it becomes apparent that we, as nurses, should become more proficient in this aspect of our communication. Many of our nursing functions depend upon our interactions with the people for whom we care. We are dependent upon our ability to communicate effectively with persons of all ages and with various backgrounds and occupations. Language makes it possible for us to talk with our patients about their concerns. Because language is symbolic, we must realize that medical and nursing language represents symbolic meanings not shared by many of our patients. This means that we must translate our symbols into meaningful language for our patients. Likewise patients do not describe their discomforts in our symbolic terms, but it is our responsibility to ascertain their meaning.

We, as nurses, have need of expressing ourselves clearly and in sentences that are complete and understandable. Many nurses have been more action oriented and have not been concerned with how they express themselves in writing or in speech. The time has arrived when we must become proficient in this latter function. If we accept the belief, and I think we should, that the primary function of language is to facilitate communication, then the primary requisite is to learn to use our language effectively.

Equally as important as learning to use our language effectively is the necessity for understanding the ways in which people communicate with each other. Nurses must be concerned with the meanings patients attempt to convey. We must not assume that situations which are usual and comfortable for us have the same meaning for patients. We must make every effort to understand the totality of the other person's situation. What is meaningful to the patient should be meaningful to us. Even the common term "surgery" connotes a different meaning to the patient than it does to us. A patient does not classify surgery as major or minor, nor does he know the specific risks that we know are involved in various kinds of surgery. My point is that their conceptions and our conceptions are frequently different. It is their conceptions on which we must focus attention, if we are to provide adequate nursing care.

BIBLIOGRAPHY

GARDNER, JOHN W. *Excellence.* New York: Harper & Row, Publishers, 1961.

HAYAKAWA, S. I. *Language, Meaning and Maturity.* New York: Harper & Row, Publishers, 1954.

———. *Language in Thought and Action.* New York: Harcourt, Brace & World, Inc., 1949.

HOEBEL, E. ADAMSON. *Man in the Primitive World.* (2d ed.) New York: McGraw-Hill Book Company, 1958.

Hoijer, Harry. "Language in Culture," Patrick and Mary Hazard, (eds.) *Language and Literacy To-Day*. Chicago: Science and Research Associates, Inc., 1965.

Huxley, Aldous. *Words and Their Meanings*. Los Angeles: The Ward Ritchie Press, 1940.

Langer, Susanne, K. *Philosophy in a New Key*. New York: The New American Library, Inc., 1951.

Larick, Stuart. "Why 'General' Semantics?," *ETC: A Review of General Semantics*, Vol. 29, No. 2, June, 1972.

Sapir, Edward. *Culture, Language and Personality*. Los Angeles: University of California Press, 1960.

Smith, Alfred G. *Communication and Culture*. New York: Holt, Rinehart & Winston, Inc., 1966.

Warfel, Harry R. *Language a Science of Human Behavior*. Cleveland: Howard Allen, Inc., 1962.

Nonverbal Communication

In the study of human communication, it is necessary to explore the many avenues of nonverbal communication. We can begin by distinguishing as nonverbal every kind of communication that does not utilize words. Although nonverbal communication might at first seem to be less effective and important than verbal, this is frequently not the case. Sometimes, in fact, the nonverbal message predominates so strongly that it completely overrides the words another person might be speaking.

An illustration of this can be seen in the following situation. You have just shaken hands with a friend, and the friend tells you on inquiry that he "feels fine." As he is telling you this, however, you notice that he quickly looks away, and that his hand feels icy cold and clammy. You also see that he exhibits a kind of "offhand" manner, and that he has steered the conversation away from himself and on to the weather. On further observation, you notice that he is standing slightly stooped, with his abdomen pulled inward. In this instance, although you heard your friend say that he felt fine, you have observed certain body manifestations, gestures, and the absence of a direct gaze that strongly communicate the opposite impression. Had you been talking to this same person on the telephone, you would not have seen these reactions. You might possibly have discerned a characteristic in the tone or pitch of his voice that you have learned to associate with the words, "I am not fine," but you could not be absolutely sure of this. By personally observing the nonverbal signs of communication, however, you were able to comprehend his total message.

Unfortunately, nonverbal signs may often go unnoticed, or may be misunderstood by many people who have not been educated to observe them. Although all of us perceive through our senses, there are variations in our perceptions which often result from our past learning and experience.

At first glance, nonverbal communication may seem to be quite simple and uncomplicated. As with all study of human beings, however, there is much more involved in it than first meets the eye. In our illustration, certain physiological signs and body gestures communicated a message, nonverbally, that did not concur with the verbal one. In this particular case, the nonverbal message was strong enough to obscure and negate the verbal message contained in the words, "I am fine." Though you might have verbally replied to the words, "I feel fine," the nonverbal messages would have very definitely altered your acceptance of the verbal message.

Charles Galloway, an educator who has made many contributions to the study of nonverbal behavior, describes it as the language of sensitivity:

> The nonverbal is indeed the language of sensitivity. It is the age-old language of lovers, that sublime communication without words. It is the language of the content, a knowing smile, an exchanged glance that tells more—much, much more than words can ever say. It is the frown that makes one feel guilty; the silent anger that emits a tenseness so real that it can almost be touched. It is that obscure, yet emphatic meaning behind the silence that thunders its message. The nonverbal is so complicated that it can convey an entire attitude, yet so simple that when a head nods or shakes everyone understands. All human relationships involve meanings that are more than words, and the nonverbal exposes the truth in these relationships.[1]

Ruesch and Kees have studied and written extensively about nonverbal behavior. Their text, *Nonverbal Communication*,[2] is one of the most comprehensive studies in this area. The text is mainly an investigation of a number of the nonverbal ways in which people communicate with one another. One feature of the book is the inclusion of a large number of photographs of people and places illustrating informal and spontaneous nonverbal methods of communication.

Ruesch and Kees point out that in our modern civilization, with the staggering number of people dealing solely in information, has come the danger of regarding abstract principles as concrete entities, and the consequent attribution of body and substance to numbers and letters. The result is a lack of clear delineation between verbal symbols and the

---

[1]Chas. M. Galloway, "Nonverbal: The Language of Sensitivity," *Theory Into Practice*, Vol. X, No. 4, October, 1971, p. 227.

[2]Jurgen Ruesch and W. Kees, *Nonverbal Communication* (Los Angeles: University of California Press, 1956).

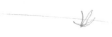

reality to which they point. If verbal and digital symbols are not repeatedly checked against the reality they signify, distortions of signification may develop. These distortions seldom occur in nonverbal language. In order to protect ourselves from modern communication technology and the distortions of propaganda, we must be careful to use words scrupulously and with integrity. Only by putting the emphasis back on the individual, with all of his personal and unique characteristics, (including nonverbal communication), can a sense of proportion and dignity be restored to human relations.

Of particular importance to nurses is Ruesch and Kees' concern that people often ignore the significance of nonverbal behavior, and give precedence to verbal behavior. Since such a wide range and variety of nonverbal actions and language systems are constantly being used and understood, Ruesch and Kees strongly believe that the separation of nonverbal from verbal communication will lead to definite misunderstandings.

Ruesch and Kees have developed a system for the classification of nonverbal forms and have delineated three distinct categories: sign language, action language, and object language.[3] These three categories provide a comprehensive, yet distinctive perspective of the nonverbal field. What we immediately notice about all forms of communication, verbal and nonverbal, is that they act directly on one or more of our five senses. Obviously, the spoken word is received by the ear, but nonverbal communication is directed at other senses as well. In fact, there are types of nonverbal communication that are directed specifically at each one of our five senses. In this chapter, we will examine the various modes of nonverbal communication in terms of the five senses which receive them.

SIGHT

Have you ever stopped to realize how much information you receive through your eyes? Of all our senses, we rely most heavily on sight for the major source of information about persons and things around us.

The eye is a remarkable recording instrument. In terms of visual acuity, it has been estimated that the normal human eye can see an object one-and-a-half feet in diameter, at a distance of forty-five miles. The primary reaction of sight is a photochemical one which takes place in the retina. Visual stimulation occurs from light which can be measured in terms of wave lengths, intensity (radiant energy), complexity (num-

_____

[3]*Ibid.*, p. 189.

ber of different wave lengths per stimulus), and saturation (number of wave lengths and particular wave lengths). In addition, the wave length is primarily a determining factor of color or hue, with each color resulting from a variation in wave length. The hue is in part dependent on the intensity of light. For example, objects at night are blurred and colorless, usually appearing in shades of grey and black. Other physiological (accommodation, convergence), and psychological cues (texture, light and shadow, relative motion) also assist us in our visual perception.[4] The physiological apparatus of the sense of sight is a highly specialized, intricate, and efficient mechanism. One of its faculties is the retention of a visual image.

Let us suppose that you go on a shopping trip to look for a dress. You look over rack after rack of dresses in various colors, fabrics, and styles. After seeing them all, you decide not to buy anything. The next day you recall one dress that you particularly liked and described it to a friend. You are able to do this because you retained a visual image of the style, the color, and the fabric. Without the ability to retain a visual image, you would have had to return to the store and look at all the dresses again.

We can revisualize a tree, our home, a blue sky, a friend's face, and a million other objects that we have seen. Of course, at times we may not have examined something thoroughly enough to imprint it, and we may need to reexamine it in detail. When we realize the tremendous advantages of sight, it is not difficult to understand the extreme deprivation of blindness, particularly for interpersonal communication.

Ruesch and Kees note that a child born blind must wait until his motor coordination is sufficiently advanced before he can explore the world by way of his hands.[5] If you have ever cared for a blind child you have doubtless observed how he learns to know you by touching you. He learns to "see" through his fingers. Although he eventually forms tactile, and sometimes auditory images, they are only a small substitute for the visual ones.

Dr. Ashley Montagu notes that in infants the senses develop in a definite sequence: (1) tactile, (2) auditory, and (3) visual. As the child approaches adolescence, the order of precedence is reversed: (1) visual, (2) auditory, and (3) tactile. He remarks that it is most important to experience tactile and auditory stimulations in the early development years, as it is through these senses we learn the "know-how" of being human; then vision becomes the most important. Dr. Montagu points out the relationship of all three senses in his statement, "Vision can only

[4]Wm. C. Morse and G. M. Wingo, *Psychology and Teaching* (New York: Scott, Foresman and Company, 1955), pp. 452-455.
[5]Ruesch and Kees, *op. cit.*, p. 179.

become meaningful on the basis of what it has felt and what it has heard."[6] This would explain how the blind gain meaning of objects even though they cannot see them.

The blind become experts in object language because all three-dimensional things are learned through tactile impressions. Words used and learned by a person, who has always been blind, do not elicit visual images. The blind are unable to fill in the numerous details that vision supplies to help us understand words and concepts. Due to absence of vision, the blind cannot learn from the actions of others—they can only learn from their own actions. Ruesch and Kees conclude their observations with the following comment: "Although the blind can inform themselves about people and things by touch, they are incapable of appreciating any two-dimensional representation, either verbal or nonverbal.[7]

Dr. Edward T. Hall states that the eyes are distance receptors, and notes that the unaided eye takes in an extraordinary amount of information within a hundred-yard radius, and that it is quite efficient for human interaction at a mile. He compares visual and auditory perception, and indicates that visual information tends to be less ambiguous and more selective than auditory information.[8] The relative efficiency of the eye and the ear is not our main concern here. What is important, however, is that we make ourselves aware of these functions in our communication process. Part of our effectiveness in providing nursing care depends upon cognizance of this avenue of communication.

If we pause to reflect, it will be obvious that we rely heavily on visual observation for the affirmation of facts or truths. The very fact that we constantly use such expressions as: "I'll believe it when I see it," "Seeing is believing," and "I want to see for myself," is clear evidence of this. It seems pertinent to remind ourselves, as nurses, that we are observed by patients even though we often operate as though this were not the case. We should be ever mindful that we do not operate behind a one-way vision screen. Perhaps nurses and patients "see" or "attend" different things. Dr. Hall believes that we all learn to "see" differently, and also asserts that men and women "attend" differently. He explains that, "these are differences which cannot be attributed to variations in visual acuity. Men and women simply have learned to use their eyes in very different ways."[9]

---

[6]Ashley Montagu, *Touching* (New York: Columbia University Press, 1971), p. 236.

[7]*Ibid.*, p. 179.

[8]Edward T. Hall, *The Hidden Dimension* (New York: Doubleday & Company, Inc., 1966), pp. 40-41.

[9]*Ibid.*, p. 65.

We should also be cognizant that patients literally see differently when lying prone in bed, and that their vision is further hindered if they wear glasses—particularly bifocals. I have had patients tell me that they couldn't find their watch, or some other object, when it was perfectly obvious to me that it was right on the table next to them. I finally recognized that the patient's range of vision was restricted by his position in bed, which prevented him from being able to see the particular article. Our communication could have failed had I not recognized his dilemma. Too often we attribute this kind of request to a bid for attention.

We verbally share our visual memories with our friends who, having seen the same or a similar thing, can readily understand. We can also observe their reaction—whether they agree, disagree, or are uninterested. We not only know their reactions by their verbal response, but also from viewing their facial expressions, gestures, and general body responses. As stated previously, we are aware that the nonverbal information we receive through our vision influences our communication with others.

Eye Contact

The eye has a unique sociological function. It promotes the union and interactions of individuals, which is a direct and pure reciprocity. A mutual glance between persons signifies a new and unique union between two persons. We seek or avoid visual contact depending on whether or not we desire this union.

A number of articles have been written by psychiatric nurses indicating the importance of "eye contact" from the patient. Their main focus has been on whether or not the patient makes eye contact with the nurse, but they have neglected to emphasize the necessity of the nurse initiating eye contact with the patient.

Teachers are also concerned with eye contact with students as a mode of communication. Mark Knapp says that students who avoid eye contact with teachers when asked a question may be saying, "I don't know the answer; I don't want to be called on, if my eyes meet the eyes of the instructor I am almost obligated to interact because I am saying the channel is open." Students get very busy with taking notes or rearranging books or papers to avoid the open channel. Knapp describes the large classroom where physical distance between teacher and student is great, eye contact can reduce the distance. However "eye contact of extended duration can also be used to indicate aggressiveness or create anxiety in others." Eye contact is decreased if dislike, competition with another, "hurt feelings," or embarrassment occur. Patients may avoid looking at the nurse if they have not followed her instructions, or they are embarrassed about their condition.[10]

Lack of eye contact occurs when the teacher is displeased with the student's performance; likewise when the nurse is displeased with a patient for demanding his medication at a scheduled hour. Teaching-learning and nursing-caring are essentially a communication process.

A student in a graduate program in psychiatric nursing examined the nonverbal behavior of selected nurses in various nurse-patient interactions. She found that nurses who, for whatever reason, wished to avoid answering the patient's question would look away, or did not look at the patient as she answered, or in some instances did not verbally answer the question. When patients involved in these interactions were queried as to "what was the behavior of the nurse," they consistently indicated whether the nurse did or did not look at them.[11]

Gestures and Body Movements

A gesture is any movement of the body or of part of the body which is used to express or emphasize ideas in conjunction with verbal expression. Gestures are a form of nonverbal language, sometimes accidental and sometimes deliberate, which are always an integral component of daily conversation. Dr. Edward Hall believes that we communicate our real feelings in our silent language—the language of behavior.[12] Ruesch and Kees believe that in interpersonal relations, gestures tend to have a more mandatory function, whereas words tend to serve a more explanatory function.[13]

Gestures usually accompany speech. As an illustration of this, let us suppose that you want someone to leave, and you say, "Get out." Often you will emphasize your statement by pointing to the door. If there is more than one door in the room, your gesture can also indicate the door you wish them to use. Many adults curl their index finger toward their body and say to a child, "Come here!" The child will understand the gesture long before he can understand the words. We all recognize the use of a raised eyebrow, a shrug of the shoulders, or a shy glance to emphasize a point.

Most of our gestures are learned by imitation of others. Generally, we are not conscious of our mannerisms, mainly because they were learned

---

[10]Mark L. Knapp, "The Role of Nonverbal Communication in the Classroom," *Theory into Practice*, Vol. X, No. 4, October, 1971, p. 246.

[11]Roseann Calvey, "Identification of Encouraging and Inhibiting Nonverbal Behaviors of Nurses in Selected Nurse-Patient Interactions and Nonverbal Behaviors Stated by Patients." Unpublished Dissertation, Catholic University, 1972, p. 27.

[12]Edward T. Hall, *The Silent Language* (Greenwich: Fawcett Publications, Inc., 1959), p. 10.

[13]Ruesch and Kees, *op. cit.*, p. 86.

out of awareness. A mother does not explicitly teach a child that a particular gesture indicates—"Come here!" The child automatically learns the meaning of such a gesture through the mother's use of it.

Within all cultures, certain gestures are adopted and children learn them as they learn other behavior patterns. I would hazard a guess that there are very few people in the United States who do not know that the index finger held perpendicular to the lips means "be quiet!" Not all people wave good-bye as we do. There are some instances, however, where a gesture has become internationally recognized. A good example of this is Churchill's famous "V" for victory sign. As a general rule, however, gestures vary markedly in meaning from one culture to another. The study of the use of gestures in communication is called Kinesics. A recent treatise in this field by Ray L. Birdwhistell advances the interesting theory that gestures, like verbal communication, can express past, present, and future time, as well as singular and plural number.[14]

"Although we have been searching for 15 years, we have found no gesture or body motion which has the same social meaning in all societies. . . . Insofar as we know, there is no body motion or gesture that can be regarded as a universal symbol. That is, we have been unable to discover any single facial expression, stance, or body position which conveys an identical meaning in all societies."[15]

It is not difficult to realize that, as nurses, we can gain valuable information about a patient's condition from his body movements and gestures. Bodily characteristics that can "communicate" a wealth of information to us include peculiarities in gait and dress, the touch of a handshake, particular mannerisms, glances and looks, skin condition and texture, the color of eyes and lips, body build, and even the most minute muscular twitching of the face, hands, ears, and eyes.

Most of us who remember the long running television program, "What's My Line," will recall that its host, John Daly, used to pull at his ear lobe when he was nervous about a particular line of questioning or some accidental blooper. Johnny Carson, on NBC's "Tonight" show, has commented on his habit of touching his nose—a habit even he was not aware of until someone mentioned it. We all know people who drum their fingers on the table, or cough or sigh deeply when they are tense. The compulsive doodler is showing behavioral signs that are clearly communicative. I have a friend who "jiggles" her foot whenever she is concerned

---

[14]Ray L. Birdwhistell, "Some Relations Between American Kinesics and Spoken American English," A. G. Smith (ed.) *Communication and Culture* (New York: Holt, Rinehart & Winston, Inc., 1966), pp. 182-189.

[15]Ray L. Birdwhistell, *Kinesics and Context* (Philadelphia: University of Pennsylvania Press, 1970), p. 81.

about something. We can see that these and many more gestures are means of expression which, when noticed and correctly interpreted, can provide a wealth of additional information that is seldom communicated by the spoken word.

It is well to note here that Ruesch and Kees see gestures as different from emotional expressions, in that "they are consciously intended for communicative exchanges, and are addressed to particular individuals." They add that if these occur when the person is alone, they are addressed "to whom it may concern."[16]

A particular note should be made regarding the importance of gestures. They often convey a different or opposite message than the verbal message they accompany. For example, you may have a great desire to meet a particular person, but if an introduction is offered, you protest verbally while nodding your head in the affirmative. If you are with an alert friend, she will probably note your real message and ignore your verbal protest. In this instance, the gesture helped you to attain your wishes. Communication thus was enhanced, because the recipient "heard" both messages. If the gesture had been ignored, faulty communication would have occurred. In general, gestures or body movements may facilitate communication. In situations where one cannot find words to express one's thoughts adequately, gestures may convey the message more successfully. Gestures generally tend to reveal a person's real desires far more than his verbal expression does.

It is important to remember that body movements and gestures are culturally learned, and are functions of our communication system. Most social psychologists and social anthropologists agree that Kinesic communication is undeniably an important part of the total process of communication.

The language of body movement found in the arts is a more formal type of communication. By this I mean that the arts generally represent a more structured aspect or agreed upon custom. General characteristics may change, but the presentation is more ordered.

Many different expressions are exhibited by the dancer through the use of the body. Some dances express harmony with the body; others denote wild paroxysms or great physical strength. The kinds of dance found in various cultures are many and varied, but each communicates something about the national culture. Pantomime is another form of nonverbal communication and those of you who have seen Marcel Marceau can appreciate the great wealth of information communicated by this

---

[16]Ruesch and Kees, *op. cit.*, p. 46.

type of nonverbal art. Clowns in the circus are another example. Some forms of dance and pantomime actually relate an entire story.

Action Signals*

A brief comment should be made about systematized actions which Ruesch and Kees indicate may be substitutes for verbal symbols or auxiliary devices for speech. These are actions whose meaning has been established by prior verbal agreement.[17] They are, therefore, not considered to be gestures in the true sense of the word. The semaphore used by our Navy, the sign language of Indians and of the deaf are examples of action signals. The particular signals developed by television directors to indicate "on the air," "two minutes remaining," etc., are other examples. Hospitals and clinics have replaced written direction signs with colored lines painted on the floor or walls, with specific colors indicating the pathways to specific areas. Though these are not yet standardized nationally, they represent a nonverbal system. Some hospitals have substituted assigned numbers which flash on and off at a central location for the verbal intercom systems used in locating physicians. Patients' call-light systems indicate "I need you!" to the nurse. All of these fall into the category of nonverbal action signals.

Facial Expression

Paul Secord writes that human physiognomy has been a focus of interest throughout recorded history. It has had a central emphasis in literature, painting and sculpture, in describing human character or being representative of the person. Secord says there are two distinctive aspects of the face presumed to be important: (1) The relative unmodifiable structure of the face, (size, shape, and arrangement of eyes, nose, and facial planes); (2) The pattern of facial expression, (relatively permanent expressions and fleeting expression).

Secord describes several determinates by which we form impressions of others from facial cues. He noted from several studies that we learn from our culture certain factors that guide our perception about the person from facial features. Various cultural perceptions regarding women, color of skin and hair, and age of the person influence the development of stereotyping of the person. Cultural factors place an emphasis on certain facial cues and give them special meaning, which does indicate there is some consensus among people of the same culture. The most common facial cue is a smile. Facial tension accounts for a second

---

*Term used by Ruesch and Kees.
[17]*Ibid.*, p. 36.

expressive characteristic of the face. However, the author notes that there is "no invariable pattern of expression accompanying specific emotions."[18]

Secord notes that people make many inferences about the person from facial features on a momentary basis, as if it were an enduring quality. We also infer by generalizing from a previous interpersonal situation to a new person. The generalization, of course, may or may not fit the new person. Other factors such as age, race, and sex are used to categorize the person, often stereotyping the person, as noted previously. Certain functional qualities of the person are perceived as an inference about the person. For example, persons with thin, compressed lips may be seen as "tight lipped." Those who have high foreheads are often said to be more intelligent. Persons who have rough skin, heavy eyebrows, or disheveled hair, may be classified as boorish, unkind, or hostile.

Secord believes that we need to examine what operates in the perceiver that influences his perception of others from his inference process. Since perception is a highly personal experience, the person may have unique categories that have personal significance for him, but are relatively ignored by others. Though studies have demonstrated that inferences are categorized according to cultural influences, studies should be made of the perceptual cognitive process.[19]

Facial expression, often used as an indicator of a person's disposition, is perhaps relied upon too consistently for accuracy. The facial expression of physical pain, for instance, is often not the same with each person, though there are some similarities among all people. Then too, a different response will occur according to the degree of physical pain, and the extent to which each person allows himself to show pain.

Some persons have been taught *not* to complain about pain. Thus, they could be experiencing pain without any facial manifestation. Irving K. Zola believes that the complaints of sick people are as much a part of their cultural background as they are a result of a particular disease. He found that response to questions about pain differed markedly in Irish and Italian patients. The Irish patients were specific and restricted in their complaints, whereas the Italian patients tended to spread and magnify theirs. Zola believes that the expression of pain, though differing in degree among various cultures, serves the same purpose in all cultures. The variations in expression arise from differences in culture, and not from a difference in the purpose of the expression.[20]

---

[18]Paul F. Secord, "Facial Features and Inference Processes in Interpersonal Perception," *Person Perception and Interpersonal Behavior,* R. Tagiuri and L. Petrullo (eds.) (Stanford: Stanford University Press, 1958), pp. 300-301.

[19]*Ibid.*, p. 301.

[20]Irving K. Zola, "Roundup of Current Research," *Trans-action,* April, 1967, p. 3.

Smiling is a facial expression that is an indicator of a person's mood. Mansfield,[21] in a study of empathic behaviors using video taped nurse-patient interviews, found that the nurses' facial expression ranged from deep concern, interest and attentive listening to smiling and shared laughter. Interest and warmth were evident in her facial expressions. The facial expression was a significant behavior which conveyed a high level of empathy. Most of us are aware and often comment positively about a person who smiles easily, such as "she is a comfortable person to be around—she always smiles," or "Even with her problems, she has a smile for others." Conversely we often remark, "She never smiles," or "It seems to be an effort for her to smile."

Although facial expressions can sometimes be excellent indicators of a patient's disposition, we must guard against making inaccurate generalizations or stereotypes which are based not on the evidence before us, but on our own past experiences with various individuals. A person who exhibits what appears to be a "grumpy" facial expression is not necessarily a "grumpy" person. You have doubtless heard the remark, "She always looks so somber, but once you get to know her, you will find she is very humorous."

We also fail to recognize that changes in facial expressions are immediate reactions. A frown from one person may not mean the same thing in another. As there are variations in all human behavior, variations of facial expression also occur from person to person. People with the proverbial "deadpan" face may make others feel uncomfortable, but their expressionless faces make them excellent poker players. Comedians strive to control their facial expression in order to highlight the verbal dialogue and reinforce the joke. Other persons, quite unconsciously, have very mobile facial expressions, and their moods are easily discernible. Almost all people register the intense emotions of fear, anger, horror, and hate in their facial expressions, so we must be constantly aware of the fact that facial expressions (or the lack of them), when interpreted correctly, are meaningful aids to communication, and are an important part of our nonverbal method of communication.

Posture

Posture can be another source of nonverbal information about a person. Mothers frequently harp at their children "to stand up straight," a posture which indicates a healthy body, (man is upright, not stooped as the animals), and a positive outlook on life. Older people, or those

---

[21]Elaine C. Mansfield, "Role Model Demonstration of Empathic Behaviors with Schizophrenic Patients in Video Taped Nurse-Patient Interviews." Unpublished Doctoral Dissertation, Catholic University, School of Nursing, 1972.

who have labored strenuously at "back-breaking" tasks, are often stooped. The erect posture of a Marine in our culture is a mark of distinction. Parents are often concerned because their adolescent son slouches. It is partly because of the implications our posture communicates about us as human beings that we need to be concerned.

The posture we achieve as adults develops gradually, and may change from youth to old age. Many factors such as occupation, body build, musculature development, health and psychological attitude about self, influence our posture. In our society, we are inclined to value an erect posture because it connotes self-respect, and is indicative of youth. Admiring comments are made of older persons, of either sex, who maintain their youthful carriage.

Abdominal surgery always alters one's posture when the first attempt is made to stand erect. Nurses invariably remonstrate "stand up straight." Their traditional respect for the upright posture suddenly emerges. One has only to experience the sensation of the unfunctioning severed abdominal muscles to appreciate the inability to comply. If the patient responds with some obscenity, the nurse should not be surprised.

Our everyday posture does provide additional information to others about ourselves. We should learn to evaluate or interpret posture correctly. We should be cautious of stereotyping, however, and consider posture in its proper relation to all other forms of communication.

Body Appearance

The clothes we wear are another source of nonverbal communication. The choice of the style, the color, and the cost of our clothing partially reveal our personal characteristics. In our society we seem to associate personal worth and prestige with our appearance. Standards of dress change from year to year, but our acceptance or rejection of the dictates of the fashion world somewhat influences other people's acceptance of us.

Our apparel conveys to a certain extent our identity, not only to ourselves but to others. Nurses working in psychiatric hospitals frequently concentrate on getting patients to dress in an appropriate manner, as though this would enhance their identity. Conversely, many nurses in general hospitals prefer that patients wear the traditional hospital gown. Perhaps this helps maintain the person's identity as a "patient." There may be other reasons for the nurses' behavior in both instances but, in either case, the clothing a patient wears by choice has some communicative value.

Closely related to our concern about clothing is the attention we give to the care of our body. In our society we spend more annually on cosmetics than we do on cancer research. Women, particularly, attempt to make themselves more attractive and acceptable by changes in their hair color or style. This seems to be a particular female trait which is not limited to women in America. Recently, men have begun to change their hair styles, and we should not overlook this in our analysis of their nonverbal expression.

Currently, our television advertisers focus upon body cleanliness, body odor, clean white teeth, and hair color as indicators for acceptance or rejection by friends, lovers, husbands, or wives. Most of the products are geared to enhancing our appearance, which infers greater acceptability.

All of these alterations in our body image may communicate ideas to others about our age, male or female identity, sense of correctness, social class, or economic status. Unfortunately, these cannot communicate information to others about our worth as a human being.

AUDITION

Almost all of our communication is received by our eyes and ears. Although we readily recognize the importance of the ear for verbal communication, less attention is paid to the function of the ears in our nonverbal communication. Physiologically, the ear is not only one sense organ but two: one function is hearing, and the other is the detection of the rotation and tilting of the head which is necessary in the maintenance of body balance. The ear has a remarkable ability to distinguish certain sounds, even against a background of chaotic noise. The outer ear, which is basically the same shape in all people, serves as a funnel for sound waves which are the necessary stimuli for audition.

Sound waves are described in terms of frequency rather than length. The three qualities of sound are dependent on the physical attributes of sound waves. They are *Pitch* (high or low), which is related to the frequency and amplitude or intensity of the sound wave; *Loudness*, measured in decibels, which is also dependent on frequency and intensity; and *Timbre* which represents a quality of sound, but is dependent upon the complexity of the stimulus. Timbre is what distinguishes tones of the same pitch. It determines the difference we hear between a note played on a violin and the same note played on an oboe. Each instrument has a fundamental tone which dominates the sound as well as overtones, which are less intense than the basic sound.[22]

Dr. Hall has found that the unaided ear is very efficient up to twenty feet. At about one hundred feet, one-way vocal communication is possible, but two-way conversation is significantly altered. The sensitivity

---

[22]Morse and Wingo, *op. cit.*, pp. 455-458.

of the normal ear for close range reception is tremendous.[23] Dr. Dominick Barbara, a psychiatrist who has worked with and studied the deaf, views the ear as an emotional instrument as well as a physical instrument of hearing. He notes that the ability to respond to sound is present at birth, and is closely related to the infant's ability to identify or separate himself from his environment. "Emotionally the ear is also the organ through which the verbal taboos and restrictions of the parents are communicated to the child. Words like 'bad,' 'dirty,' 'naughty,' etc., used to discipline the child through the intonation and intensity of their utterance, are all transmitted to the child's psyche through the ear."[24] Thus the ear serves a double function in communication: physiologically for the reception of sound, and psychologically for the perception of attitudes associated with words.

Listening

The act of listening requires more than just the comprehension of words spoken by the other person. Francis Chisholm describes his concept of listening in the following manner:

> The relation between what the speaker says and what the listener hears is not a one-to-one symmetrical relationship. It has characteristics which make it necessary to classify it as some kind of asymmetrical relationship. No matter how attentively or accurately I listen, I cannot get all your nuances, the connotations words have for you, the emphases and reservations you have, etc. What I hear is less than what you have said. But it is also more than what you said: No matter how "objective" I may be, I cannot entirely avoid projecting my "understanding" of the words you send me. You say it in your frame of assumptions: I hear it in mine. The two may not be incommensurable (we may speak the "same" language and have the "same" interests); but, as the telephone engineers would say, the line has noise and distortion. But many people behave as if the relation between "what he says" and "what I hear" were one of simple equality; i.e., a symmetrical relationship. (The evidence is too overwhelming to require "proof." Have you ever been misquoted. Have you ever found yourself elaborately refuting something which, it develops, the other fellow never said?)[25]

Hayakawa supports the requirements of listening in the following statement:

> Listening requires entering actively and imaginatively into the other fellow's situation and trying to understand a frame of reference different from your own. This is not always an easy task.[26]

---

[23]Hall, *The Hidden Dimension, op. cit.,* p. 41.
[24]Dominick A. Barbara, *The Art of Listening* (Springfield: Charles C Thomas, Publisher,1958), p. 23.
[25]Francis P. Chisholm, "A New Kind of Comprehension Test," *Journal of Communication,* Vol. 5, Fall, 1955, p. 84.
[26]S. I. Hayakawa, "How to Attend a Conference," *ETC: A Review of General Semantics,* Autumn, 1955, p. 7.

The information we receive through the ear is completely different from that which we receive through sight. Dr. Joost Meerloo provides a significant differentiation in the following comment: "The ear provides a more highly differentiated world of impressions than does the eye. Our sound world is related to the world of rhythm and time. . . . The spoken sound disappears; we can never come back to it, and we cannot verify it again and again. The visual picture, on the other hand, is imbued with reality."[27]

Accepting the premise offered by Chisholm, there is reason to concern ourselves with the process of listening. Simeon Potter comments on the interrelationship between listening and talking:

> Communication is ever two-way. Listening is the other half of talking. Listening well is no less important than speaking well and it is probably more difficult. Could you listen to a 45 minute discourse without once allowing your thoughts to wander? Good listening is an art that demands the concentration of all your mental facilities. In general, people in the western world talk better than they listen. Competition in our way of life encourages "self-expression" even in those who have little or nothing to express! While ostensibly listening to a discussion, many people are inwardly framing a form of words that will both stun the assembly and lay low their opponents.[28]

It seems pertinent to make the distinction between hearing and listening at this time so that we can more fully comprehend the meaning of listening. "To hear" means specifically to become aware of sounds. It is essentially a passive thing, occurring automatically when sound waves stimulate the auditory nerves. "To listen" requires one to make an active, conscious effort to attend closely to the auditory stimuli. The distinction between the two words lies in "the conscious effort" required for listening, which makes it more active than just hearing a sound.

Listening as an art requires discipline and concentration as prerequisites. Concentration requires us to remove distractions that interfere with listening. Dr. Barbara sees the effectual listener as a person with an open mind, who attempts to find something interesting in what is being said. He describes the ineffectual listener as being on the defensive, planning rebuttals or questions which may embarrass or belittle the other person. The same author includes comprehension as an important factor in effective listening. Comprehension involves the attempt to understand and grasp the true idea or meaning of what is heard. Dr. Barbara reminds us that we speak about one hundred and twenty-five words per minute,

---

27J. A. M. Meerloo, *Conversation and Communication* (New York: International Universities Press, 1952), p. 18.

28Simeon Potter, "Language and Society," Patrick and Mary Hazard (eds.) *Language and Literacy Today* (Chicago: Science Research Associates, Inc.), 1965, p. 6.

but that we think four times that fast. He says, "it is what we do with this extra time that makes us either good or poor listeners."[29]

Listening ability has for many years been considered an essential ingredient for providing "good" nursing care, and yet Ida Orlando has recently noted that one patient told his story ten times without ever having it comprehended by the nurse.[30] An examination of a variety of nursing publications revealed that nurses are aware of the need to listen, but patients continue to report that "the nurse is too busy to listen." It would be a rare event if a patient were this direct with a nurse. Patients generally have the expectation that the nurse will listen and it would not be polite to remind her to do so.

The need for listening is not confined to the nurse-patient situation. Schools of education are aware of the need for students to listen efficiently. Research on the hearing ability of students as well as listening retention has been conducted on various educational levels. Educators have substituted the seminar for lectures, because students cannot concentrate for long periods of time on the spoken word, and there is more involvement in a seminar discussion.

To be an effective listener, Combs and Snygg speak of "intent listening" to convey the active process required for listening. Thus to listen, a person must attend. Many of us hear only what we wish to hear. Dr. H. S. Sullivan has labelled this "selective inattention." That is, we pick out what we wish to hear and discard the rest. Whatever the reasons may be, the end result is a limiting of communication.

It seems that if we, as nurses, are to listen efficiently and intently to those persons in our care, we must be cognizant of the conscious effort and concentration this entails. Even then we cannot grasp all the meaning a person intends to convey. This is in part due to our varying ability to understand a person's words. Our interpretation of the message may sometimes be wholly inaccurate.

What does this mean operationally? There are no ground rules which govern how an individual listens to another individual. It would be possible to list a number of facial expressions, or describe a specific pose, or note that silence is required while the other person speaks, but these could easily result in mannerisms to be learned. How one listens is highly individual, and the behavior a person assumes when listening depends on his personal feelings, beliefs, how he feels about the other person and about himself. There is no right or wrong way to listen—either you listen, half listen, or don't listen at all. We have tended in the past to

[29]Barbara, *op. cit.*, p. 4.
[30]Ida Jean Orlando, *The Dynamic Nurse-Patient Relationship* (New York: G. P. Putnam's Sons, 1961), p. 57.

formulate specifics which included awareness of the tone of voice which may indicate a feeling (momentary or prolonged) of silence, or a perceived difficulty in the use of words to express the message. We must listen to the other person's words, and we must be constantly aware that their meaning for him may be different than for us. We can and should supplement the spoken word with an accurate understanding of the nonverbal communication that the patient uses as he speaks. It should be clear that nonverbal communication, when adequately received and understood, can be of great help to us in understanding a patient's message.

Hayakawa suggests the following may occur if we take time to listen: (a) we may learn something we never knew before; (b) the other person may modify his statement, as he proceeds to explain his experience; (c) communication does occur between us, and he may listen to us; and (d) both persons may profit from the conversation.[31]

To be deprived of the ability to hear alters life completely. We gradually lose our ability to hear as we grow older. Some of you have become aware of the difficulty your grandparents have in using the telephone, often because they cannot hear as distinctly as they once did. The person who is born deaf is cut off from innumerable events of life. The deaf cannot utilize the various audible danger signals like the fire alarm, the clanging of the train signal, or the ambulance siren. Many deaf patients are afraid to go to sleep at night in the hospital because they would not be able to hear the fire alarm. In addition, they miss the song of the birds and the various voice tones of their friends. Those of us who do not have this impairment should recognize that the ability to listen is a rare gift. Nurses have long considered this an essential function for understanding the patient.

How many of us stop to think about the communication problem of the totally deaf person. In a recent study, "Meeting the Health Needs of the Totally Deaf," by Harte, Furfey, Douglas, and Walsh, it is pointed out that the hearing handicapped can have real problems when they are in need of medical diagnosis and treatment. The study also showed that nurses were unaware that a severe hearing loss could present problems in communication. The nurses "seemed unaware of the fact that the socialization problem for the deaf patient entering the hospital was far more difficult than for the hearing person, because of the communication barrier." The nurses in this study tended to label those with severe hearing loss as "difficult" patients.

---

[31]S. I. Hayakawa, *Language in Thought and Action* (New York: Harcourt, Brace & World, Inc., 1949), p. 238.

Another finding of the study has direct implications for nurses. It was found that some deaf persons were unwilling to admit they did not understand their physician's instructions for the treatment of their child's illness. Consequently, unless they had professional help from another source, such as the Public Health Nurse, they were liable to become confused and emotionally disturbed, and perhaps follow a treatment quite different from that prescribed by the physician.[32] It is easy to understand that a person with a hearing loss would not wish to remind the nurse or physician that they are handicapped. One would expect that the professional would take the initiative in seeing that the deaf parent understood. Ruesch and Kees remind us that "the deaf are more unfortunate than the blind, because the loss of hearing isolates them almost completely from others."[33] Dr. Barbara concurs and notes that this isolation may lead to psychosis, though this is rarely true for the blind.[34]

Silence

Along with listening, we must also take into consideration the act of being silent. It is necessary to be silent if we wish to listen to another person. Many people are not good listeners for this very reason. A good listener, as previously noted, must attend closely to what the other person is saying, which without silence could not occur. Dominick Barbara describes the effective listener as one who *uses* silence with as much eagerness as he uses talk.

It is becoming increasingly necessary for nurses to be more precise in their use of words when they describe patients' perceptions. Recently, a group of nurses developed a list of sixteen words describing kinds of pain. These were to become part of a computerized admission form. Prior to this, they had not realized there were these many descriptive terms relevant to pain. Physicians reported that these descriptions greatly assisted them in assessing patients' conditions.

Just as we have tended to use the one word "pain" to describe all kinds of pain, we have also been inclined to use the one word "silent" to describe various kinds of silent behavior. We should be aware that there are four other words which are synonyms for the word silent and which, if understood, would better describe certain variations of silent behavior. The word *taciturn* applies to a person who is habitually uncommunicative. A *reserved* person implies a habitual disposition to be withdrawn in speech and self-restrained in manner. The word *reticent* implies a

---

[32]Thomas J. Harte, P. H. Furfey, A. M. Douglas, *et al.*, "Meeting the Health Needs of the Totally Deaf," unpublished report, Department of Social Research, The Catholic University of America, Washington, D. C., 1964, pp. 1-27.

[33]Ruesch and Kees, *op. cit.*, p. 179.

[34]Barbara, *op. cit.*, pp. 26-28.

disinclination, sometimes temporary as from embarrassment, to express one's feelings or impart information. The *secretive* person is one who suggests the furtive or evasive reticence of one who conceals things unnecessarily.[35] If we could learn to describe our patients more accurately, we could refine our observation and prevent the "lumping" of people into a restrictive category. Because of this, we tend to lose our ability to discriminate, and we develop stereotypes about those who are silent.

All of us know people, including nurses, who have great difficulty in tolerating the silence of others. Nurses frequently complain when a patient doesn't talk. The person who rarely speaks in a group often produces concern and a certain amount of uncomfortableness in the other members. We have all attended discussion groups interspersed with periods of silence, during which members fidgit, yawn, or revert to various mannerisms until speech is resumed.

To many persons, silence is frightening and something to be avoided. I once had a friend who could not tolerate silence at mealtime. From a childhood experience, silence at mealtime was an ominous clue to disagreement between mother and father. She talked for talk's sake, a sort of compulsive warding off of trouble. In the early 1900s parents frequently reared their children according to the old adage, "Children should be seen, but not heard," an attitude that applied both at home and outside. It is a rarity to hear the phrase today, since our values toward silence have been altered both for children and adults.

For centuries, silence indicated wisdom and various other positive values. These values, however, have diminished with time. Many people see only the negative aspect of silence: a disapproval, lack of accord, or intense hate. Many cartoons in our society picture the husband as the silent, and the wife as the talkative partner. The wife is rebuked or censored for her prattle, and the husband's silence is accepted as an appropriate response.

It seems that we receive confusing messages regarding the value of silence. Silence has generally not been sanctioned by psychotherapists. Silence was seen by psychiatrists as a patient's resistance to dealing with his problems. Dr. Ferreira noted in 1964 that silence in psychotherapy was discouraged even by more or less authoritarian means. With the advent of psychoanalysis, silence came to be recognized as symbolic of various pathologies. These views are no longer seen as valid, and it is more common now to treat silence like any other happening that characterizes human behavior and emotional life.[36] Dr. Barbara describes quali-

---

[35]*Webster's New World Dictionary* (New York: The World Publishing Company, 1957), p. 1357.

[36]N. J. Ferreira, "On Silence," *American Journal of Psychotherapy*, Vol. 18, January, 1964, pp. 109-114.

tatively the range of silence, from an appearance of coldness, sternness, defiance, disapproval, or condemnation, to calmness, warmth, approval, humility, or excuse.[37] It is necessary to understand both the positive and the negative aspects of silence, so that silence can become less threatening. When we do, we will readily see the benefits to be derived.

Dr. Sidney J. Baker has identified two main forms of interpersonal silence. They are: (a) positive silence, characterized by psychic equilibrium and reciprocal identification between partners (lovers or intimate friends); and (b) negative, tense silence, characterized by acute psychic disequilibrium and nonidentification between partners (anger, hate, or fear). He believes that neither form of silence is completely cognitive nor completely emotional in character, but that the ego functions are more dominant in positive silence and more unconscious in negative silence. Dr. Baker believes, however, "that the unconscious aim behind all speech is silence." He believes that we attempt to achieve psychic equilibrium, contentment, and tranquility, and that we constantly strive, through speech, to discharge psychic energy in order to become silent.[38] This is indeed a different and interesting view to consider.

Silence can and does afford relief to some people. Consider the mother of several small children who welcomes bedtime for the youngsters as a relief from the noise they make. Have you ever visited the riveting section of a large industrial plant and hurried through to escape the deafening sounds? Many of us who live in large metropolitan centers enjoy the serenity of the forests away from the multitudinous sounds of the city's activity. Radio, television, air-conditioners, and all the electrical appliances that hum and buzz, offer a constant barrage to our ears. The myriad sounds of the automobile and the whine of jet engines can be heard miles away from their origin. The quietness of a lake cottage or a mountain cabin offers relief from these daily encroachments on the ears of modern man. Modern society does not offer many escapes. There are even fewer "quiet zone" signs around our hospitals today. Our public libraries offer one of the very few remaining sanctuaries of quiet.

We are becoming less and less concerned with the need for less auditory stimulation as an aid to rehabilitation. Recent studies have shown that physiologically our bodies should receive less auditory stimulation than our society allows. Dr. Barbara indicates that extra energy is required to adapt to sounds, and that a person must learn what to expect, and how to interpret what he hears. If the person has inadequate re-

---

[37]Barbara, *op. cit.*, p. 175.
[38]Sidney J. Baker, "The Theory of Silences," *Journal of General Psychology*, Vol. 53, 1955, pp. 145-167.

serves, he may begin to show fatigue, digestive disturbances, weight loss, anxiety, and other symptoms of maladaptation to stress.[39]

We know that continual exposure to certain sounds causes a loss of hearing acuity. It is for this reason that all riveters are required to have a hearing test at regular intervals. It is sometimes forgotten that silence is a necessary ingredient for both physical and psychological health. There are many situations in each of our lives when silence serves as a curative force. When we experience grief over the death of a loved one, or grief from rejection by another, we say, "I can't talk about it." Such a strong emotional experience frequently cannot be expressed in words, and silence allows us time to adapt or cope with our feelings.

Dr. Barbara posits that through the constructive use of silence, we weave stronger ties with others and develop deeper feelings than words can possibly achieve. Furthermore, by means of silent contemplation, we can view others as they actually are, and not as we wish they were. Through silence we are able to dissolve the barriers of our tensions and cautiousness, and exchange instead the integration and unification of our inner energies toward self-realization and inner communication. He also emphasizes the use of silence to help us know ourselves more accurately, though he admits this is difficult because of man's increasing aversion to being alone with himself. He notes that for some persons, the fear of being alone with silence is so intense that any activity, regardless of purpose, is preferable.[40]

Too many people associate aloneness with loneliness! We live in a hurly-burly society that values enterprising, gregarious behavior, instant wisdom, and instant decisions. Contemplative thinking and planning are no longer viewed as a means of accomplishing our tasks, or as fitting for our daily associations with others. If we are to develop compatibility with our fellowman, we must be willing to listen, to discard our prejudices and preconceived ideas, and to learn the value that silence affords.

We should not forget that man is responsible for the existence of silences in nature as a result of his greed and lack of appreciation for the order of the universe. Allen Eckert, author of the *Silent Sky*,[41] vividly recreates man's extinction of the passenger pigeon. It is a shockingly vivid description of the eradication of more than a million birds that has contributed to an incredible silence in the world. A similar example is the account in the *Silent Spring* by the late Rachael Carson of another of mankind's atrocities. She describes man's war against nature with chem-

---

[39]Dominick A. Barbara, *Psychological and Psychiatric Aspects of Speech and Hearing* (Springfield: Charles C Thomas, 1960), p. 122.
[40]Barbara, *The Art of Listening, op. cit.*, p. 179.
[41]Allen Eckert, *The Silent Sky* (Boston: Little, Brown and Company, 1965).

icals created for use in killing insects, weeds, rodents, and other organisms. Man has assaulted his environment by contamination of the air,
earth, rivers, and seas with lethal materials. Not only has the use of
these chemicals killed millions of birds, but humans as well. Miss Carson
described the ominous silence resulting from the use of these chemicals
in the following quotation: "Over increasingly large areas of the United
States, spring now comes unheralded by the return of the birds, and the
early mornings are strangely silent where once they were filled with the
beauty of bird song."[42]

The following poem expresses some values of silence.

SILENCE

Silence widens spaces,
Fills places,
Brings graces,
Rests in greatness;
Invisible, yet Manifest;
Intangible, yet felt;
Extending far off, yet intimate.

Silence weaves together
Love, truth, and beauty.
Silence heals in grief,
Reveals in love,
Strengthens in courage.
Silence is born in love
Silence dies in tears.

Helen Manock[43]

TOUCH

Another avenue of nonverbal communication is the sense of touch.
Little significance has been given to this mode of communication by
nurses, though it is frequently a component of nursing care. In recent
years, less emphasis has been placed on backrubs and bathing as a source
of physical comfort. Some nurses frown on giving a backrub to a patient
who is ambulatory. The need for a backrub has mainly been based on
prevention of decubiti or abrasions, rather than on soothing or stimulating the nerve innervations of the skin.

---

[42]Rachel Carson, *The Silent Spring* (Boston: Houghton Mifflin Company, 1962),
p. 103.
[43]Helen Manock, "Silence," *Perspectives in Psychiatric Care,* Vol. 2, No. 2, 1964,
p. 45.

In psychiatric nursing, a taboo has been placed on female nurses giving a backrub to a male patient, because this has been interpreted as sexually stimulating. Recently, Mercer tried to determine if touch constituted a comfort or a threat in the care of the mentally ill person. In reviewing both pros and cons, she concluded that by establishing a relationship with the patient through various interactions, the freedom to touch or not to touch the patient will evolve from the relationship.[44]

James Gibson distinguishes between active touch (tactile scanning) and passive touch (being touched). He indicates that without the help of the sense of sight, we are more accurate (95%) in distinguishing objects by active touch than by passive touch (49%).[45] We know, for example, that tactile sensitivity differs from one location of the body to another. The particular location of the touch would doubtless alter the response of the person touched—a situation that is in part culturally determined. For example, in our culture a woman's response to a touch on the arm is generally different than her response to a touch on the breast. Dr. Lawrence K. Frank notes that the "lightness or heaviness of touch" indicates a quality of the message, and the recipient may respond largely to the intent or quality of the touch.[46]

Ashley Montagu, an anthropologist, in his book *Touching* indicates his interest in the skin, not just as an organ of the body, but in the manner in which tactile experience or its lack affects the development of behavior; hence, "the mind of the skin."[47]

Dr. Frank views touch and tactile experiences of the individual as highly significant in human communication. He maintains that tactile sensitivity is one of the primary modes of communication and orientation. In many interpersonal relations tactile "language" communicates more fully than vocal language. The inherited responses to signals of warm, cold, pain, and pressure comprise the tactile responses. It is through touch that we become orientated to the spatial dimensions of the world and people. We can readily see, therefore, that the skin as an organ of communication is highly complex and versatile.

Many motor activities involving the hands, fingers, and feet are guided by touch. Dr. Frank says that we often neglect the significance of the various orifices and sphincters, such as the mouth and lips, the anus and perineum, the genitals, the nose, and eyelids, as organs for tactile re-

---

[44]Lianne S. Mercer, "Touch: Comfort or Threat?" *Perspectives in Psychiatric Care,* Vol. 4, 1966, pp. 20-25.

[45]James Gibson, "Observations on Active Touch," *Psychological Review,* Vol. 69, November, 1962, p. 486.

[46]Lawrence K. Frank, "Tactile Communication," *ETC: A Review of General Semantics,* Vol. 16, Autumn, 1958, pp. 39-44.

[47]Ashley Montagu, *Touching* (New York: Columbia University Press, 1971), p. 1.

ception. Dr. Frank sees the infant's tactile experiences as playing an integral role in his personality development, and an essential role in the development of the many forms of symbolic recognition and response necessary for later learning and maturation. He believes these are learned by cultural patterning of symbolic processes. That is, the parents in any given culture activate or limit the infant's tactile communication by traditional patterns and relationships.[48]

Dr. Edward T. Hall states further that there are cultural differences in the use of touch in social and business conversation. In the United States, the handshake is most commonly used between men. In Latin America, the left hand is placed on the other man's shoulder during the handshake. A more intimate greeting involves an embrace. In North America, this practice would be embarrassing and would inhibit communication. The Japanese, on the other hand, restrict physical contact even more than we Americans. They would consider the placement of the hand on the shoulder of another as a humiliating gesture.[49]

In the United States, we measure the warmth or sincerity of a person by his handshake. A hearty firm grip indicates the person is sincere and is happy to see us or meet us. The "limp" handshake generally denotes a cool reception or a cold personality. The handshake is thus a helpful clue to a person's attitude about himself and other people.

Joost A. M. Meerloo notes that the handshake originated as a sign that two people were without weapons, and meant no harm to each other. The act of handshaking today has become a means of communicating how we feel about each other, and may still represent a silent, magical communication device—a moment when we take each other in.[50] We are all aware of the variations that we experience in receiving a handshake—variations of pressure, duration, awkwardness, or the seductive squeeze. Our initial handshake with a person represents, in part, our ease or discomfort in meeting an unknown person.

One other aspect of touch which demonstrates the scope of this sense is the adaptation made by the blind in learning to read braille.

Dr. Hall in his recent book, *The Hidden Dimension*, classifies touch as an immediate receptor. Touch includes the sensations we receive from the skin, membrane, and muscles. The skin, as the chief organ of touch, is also "sensitive to heat gain and loss, both radiant and conducted heat." Thus, the skin is both an immediate and a distance receptor. Dr. Hall

[48]Frank, *op. cit.*, pp. 209-255.
[49]Edward T. Hall and Wm. F. Whyte, "Intercultural Communication: A Guide to Men of Action," *Human Organization*, Vol. 19, Spring, 1960, pp. 5-12.
[50]Joost A. M. Meerloo, "Greeting as a Trial Approval," *Archives of General Psychiatry*, Vol. 15, September, 1966, pp. 256-259.

also notes that "touch is the most personally experienced of all sensations." He says that although we have a great deal of knowledge about the skin as a receptor, we have failed to grasp the significance of active touch in our environment.[51]

Particularly important for nurses working with infants in the nursery is Dr. Montagu's description of "Tender Loving Care." During the nineteenth century more than half the infants in their first year of life died from a disease called *Marasmus*, a Greek word meaning "wasting away." The death rate for infants in foundling institutions throughout the United States was nearly 100 percent even into the second decade of the twentieth century. Through the work of several pediatricians it was discovered that with adequate mothering these infants did not die. Montagu reports:

> What the child requires if it is to prosper, it was found, is to be handled, and carried, and caressed, and cuddled, and cooed to, even if it isn't breast fed. It is the handling, the carrying, the caressing, the cuddling that we would here emphasize, for it would seem that even in the absence of a great deal else, there are the reassuringly basic experiences the infant must enjoy if it is to survive in some semblance of health. Extreme sensory deprivation in other respects, such as light and sound, can be survived, as long as the sensory experiences at the skin are maintained.[52]

Doubly important, as stated by Montagu, is that the child establishes its first communicative relationship through its kinesic sense. Everybody is born with this kinesic sense—the evidence is—experimental, observational, experiental and anecdotal. Dr. Montagu describes the function of the nose, breathing, the lips and function of the mouth, touching and feeling, grasping and learning, as important aspects of the maturation of the child. He makes more explicit than Dr. Frank the necessary actions of the mother in the care of the child. We, as nurses, have much to learn about the significance of touch as an essential component of nursing care. Our ministrations should include more than "cooling the fevered brow." There is particular need for a recognition of the communication properties of touch, and a need for nursing research in this area.

GUSTATION

Of all our senses, taste has less direct influence on our communication than our other senses. The sense of taste is closely allied with the sense of smell, so much so that without it we are unable to taste various

---

[51]Hall, *The Hidden Dimension, op. cit.,* pp. 40-59.
[52]Montagu, *op. cit.,* p. 84.

foods. We all know that when we have a cold and as a result of nasal congestion, food either tastes differently or is entirely flavorless. Certain very strong disagreeable odors can cause nausea and vomiting.

Some psychiatric patients seem to have a distortion of taste; they state that their food and drink tastes like poison. Since it is highly unlikely that they have tasted poison previously, they must experience a change in taste and construe this as a change in the food rather than in their ability to taste. Some people believe that this is due to a change in thinking—a projection. Of this we cannot be certain. Many patients who have experienced this will tell you later that their food actually tasted differently at that time.

We frequently describe women with phrases associated with taste. We say, "She's a sweet person," or "She's a honey." Certain characteristics of people become associated with specific foods, such as, "He's a ham" or "Don't be such a goose." If we hear an unlikely tale, we say, "That was strictly corn" or "He was so corny." All of these convey certain positive or negative connotations about the person.

The gustatory receptors are located mainly on the surface of the tongue, although a few are found in the mucous membrane of the mouth and throat. There are certain conspicuous taste sensations: sweet, bitter, sour, salt. Some parts of the tongue are more sensitive to one sensation than to another. The taste buds, as these receptors are named, readily adapt to stimulation. One taste may heighten sensitivity to another—a contrast effect—or may lessen the sensitivity to another—neutralization.[53] Just as our clothing reflects individual and social characteristics about us as a person or a nation, the food we eat and the liquor we drink are further indications about us. Rice and fish have long been a staple food of the Orient, corn and beans in Mexico; various spices are abundant in Italian foods, and wine is a part of every Frenchman's diet. These are but a few of the hundreds of variations peculiar to a given society.

Endless variations regarding particular likes and dislikes of certain foods occur with individuals and in geographical areas. Certain foods are thought of as foods to be served at breakfast; others are considered sandwich foods. In part, these differences are culturally determined, and in some nations they are determined by geographical conditions. Some lands can be tilled. Others, like Alaska with its short growing seasons, must depend mainly on animal food. More than any other nation in the world, we are less dependent on geographical determinants as food regulators, since our ability to transport food from one part of the country to another allows us to obtain almost any kind of food available, as long

---

[53]Morse and Wingo, *op. cit.*, pp. 461-462.

as we have the money to purchase it. We must recognize that tastes for certain foods are often culturally determined, and are not just individual eccentricities.

For us, the manner in which we serve our food communicates our social and economic status. There are a few people who still use their fingers instead of utensils to pick up their food. For the most part, however, we eat with silver, or more recently, with stainless steel. Likewise, we spend a great deal of time choosing china, glassware, etc. All of these utensils signify wealth, genteelness, or a current fad which we display when partaking of food. When we entertain others we generally use our best china, linens, and silver, and serve special foods, not only to convey our desire to please our guests, but also, in many instances, to display our "taste" in pattern or design, as well as our economic standing. These all have high communicative value in our society. Just as some foreigners cannot enjoy our beef, or drink our martinis, we have difficulty accepting the tea of the English in place of our coffee.

The hours of eating comprise an additional variation from one country to another. As Frances MacGregor pointed out, there is nothing biologically right about three meals a day, but it has been culturally determined in America. Unfortunately, we in America are prone to consider other cultural patterns as "wrong," if they do not coincide with ours. We forget that they are right for them. In part, this attitude toward the customs of other nations has earned us the title of the "ugly American." The label communicates our general disrespect for the cultural rights of others.

OLFACTORY

The sense of smell, along with vision and audition, is also a distance receptor. Very little is known about our olfactory sense, and there seems to be less interest in it than in our other senses. Smell is perceived in the olfactory epithelium, an area about 2 cm. square, located on either side of the nasal passages. The receptors for smell are easily fatigued after several minutes of continuous stimulation by a specific odor. Once fatigued, the receptors lose their ability to recognize the odor. If, however, another odor is immediately presented, the fatigue to the first stimulus does not impair the sensing of the second stimulus.[54] This phenomena is clearly evidenced by nurses. Visitors entering a hospital are immediately aware of the odors of various disinfectants, ether, and assorted cleaning compounds. Nurses are not generally aware of these odors,

---

[54]Stanley W. Jacob and C. A. Francone, *Structure and Function in Man* (Philadelphia: W. B. Saunders Company, 1965), p. 276.

since their receptors have become fatigued, and have lost the ability to recognize the odors.

Many attempts have been made to classify odors, but little agreement exists among experimenters. Each substance causes its own particular sensation. A multitude of distinct odors can be recognized, and individual odors in mixed smells can be distinguished. There are several theories regarding the physiology of smell, but again, there is disagreement. The main point of agreement is that the necessary stimulus is chemical in nature.

How does olfaction affect our communication? Edward T. Hall believes it could be vitally important in our relationships, but that we Americans have deprived ourselves of many olfactory stimuli. He bases his beliefs on the way Europeans differ from us in their acceptance of odors as a part of daily living. For example, we have very few of the city odors that are found in a typical French city—spices, fresh vegetables, freshly plucked fowl, clean laundry, and the odors of outdoor cafés. These odors, he believes, provide a sense of life, and assist us in locating ourselves in space.[55] The odors of our cities, unfortunately, are predominately the smell of gasoline or smoke from industrial plants. The odors of jet combustion are overwhelming, even when one is aboard the airliner.

There is one small city in the United States where gasoline is not the primary odor. That is Durham, North Carolina, where the pleasant aroma of fresh tobacco pervades the air as you enter the city.

We in America tend to associate adverse personal characteristics with smell. If we are being derogatory we say, "You stink." Our early New England fathers believed "cleanliness was next to godliness." Although more than odor was implied in this statement, we have come to associate "dirty" with a bad odor.

Adamson Hoebel, in discussing criteria of racial superiority, says that body odor has been one of the popular criteria. The white race has long used the body odor of the negro race as a reason for discrimination. Dr. Hoebel indicates that the Chinese find the smell of the white race quite distinguishable and distasteful.[56] Human perspiration does emit different odors, but we have very little information about the biochemistry of perspiration. Dr. Hoebel concludes that distinctive body odors may be an inherent racial trait, but there is no evidence that one odor is superior to another. The French are much less concerned about body odor, and French men believe that by bathing so frequently we American women lessen the ardor of the opposite sex.

---

[55]Hall, *The Hidden Dimension, op. cit.,* pp. 40-41.
[56]Adamson E. Hoebel, *Man in the Primitive World* (New York: McGraw-Hill Book Company, 1958), p. 141.

Olfaction plays a very important part in Arab life, as reported by Dr. Hall. The Arab enjoys good smells, and finds pleasure in smelling his friends. Arabs do not attempt to eliminate body odors, but strive to enhance them. Arabs distress Americans because they consistently breathe on people when they talk. For an Arab, to deny a friend your breath is to act ashamed. The American is more concerned with direct eye contact. The Arab will not hesitate to tell another that he has "bad breath," whereas we tend to consider it an insult.[57] Apparently both Americans and Arabs want to smell "nice," but the main difference is in our communication which reflects our attitude about body odor.

We have various expressions related to smell, such as, "I smell a rat," indicating something may be wrong in a situation. Another, "Don't sniffle" or "Don't be nosey" refer to adverse personal characteristics. It is interesting that we coin verbal phrases involving our sensory apparati to communicate more succinctly.

Physical deterioration of bodily tissue is frequently accompanied by a disagreeable odor. A patient who has such a condition may suffer from the nonverbal facial expressions exhibited by nurses caring for him. It is difficult not to react to these odors, but by so doing, the patient may feel we do not wish to care for him. It would be more helpful to the patient to indicate verbally that you know the odor must be distressful to him. Such a comment may help you reduce your nonverbal expression and allow the patient to feel you are more concerned about his reaction than your own.

Since our society has great concern about odors, nurses must become more cognizant of how they verbally and nonverbally deal with various odors associated with their patients.

SPACE

For this particular topic, I am indebted to Edward T. Hall, anthropologist, whose study in this area is unique. I have included it because this dimension—space—has many implications for nursing. Unfortunately, I am able to mention only a fraction of the wealth of material he presents in *The Hidden Dimension*.[58]

Dr. Hall originated the term *Proxemics* to describe the "interrelated observations and theories of man's use of space as a specialized elaboration of culture." Dr. Hall's research relative to space is centered on the

---

[57]Hall, *The Hidden Dimension, op. cit.,* p. 49.
[58]Edward T. Hall, *The Hidden Dimension* (New York: Doubleday & Company, Inc., 1966). Used by permission of the Doubleday & Company, Publishers, British Empire rights granted by Lurton Blassingame.

idea that communication constitutes the core of culture and of life itself. His research indicates that, "people from different cultures not only speak different languages but what is more important, *inhabit different sensory worlds.*" His purpose is to bring to our awareness man's use of space—the space that he maintains between himself and others—including that which he builds around him in his home or in his office. The environment which man produces alters his interactions with others. More significantly, Dr. Hall states that, *"Man and his environment participate in molding each other.*" He says that in our culture we have developed very specific spatial distances between persons, which depend upon the situation and the message to be conveyed. One common source of information about the distance separating two people is the loudness of voice. From his observations of shifts in voice in social settings, he observed four main distances: intimate, personal, social, and public (each with a close and far phase). How people feel toward each other, and what they are doing at the time they are together, are decisive factors in the distances used. He describes in detail the various activities that accompany each of the classifications.

The concept of how we use space is particularly important today, as Dr. Hall indicates, because the world's populations are crowding into cities, and builders and speculators are packing people into vertical filing-boxes—both offices and dwellings—and yes, even hospitals. With less space available, stress increases; sensitivity and crowding rises, and people get more and more on edge. They need more space, but less is available. Nurses should become aware of the spatial distances they set for patients, and how they invade the territories of patients. The way in which we order space in our hospitals influences the behavior of patients. Dr. Hall describes a study done in a large health and research center in Saskatchewan, Canada, which demonstrated that the structuring of semifixed features (furniture in the dayroom and cafeteria) did have a profound effect on the behavior of patients.

We have now seen how the various senses play an important role in our verbal and nonverbal communication. How we will make use of the various kinds of communication available to us depends in part on our ability to perceive the data. In the next chapter, we shall discuss some of the complex problems of perception.

BIBLIOGRAPHY

BAKER, SIDNEY J. "The Theory of Silences." *Journal of General Psychology*, Vol. 53, 1955.
BARBARA, DOMINICK A. *The Art of Listening.* Springfield: Charles C Thomas, Publisher, 1958.

————. *Psychological and Psychiatric Aspects of Speech and Hearing.* Springfield: Charles C Thomas, Publisher, 1960.

BIRDWHISTELL, RAY L. "Some Relations Between American Kinesics and Spoken American English," A. G. Smith (ed.) *Communication and Culture.* New York: Holt, Rinehart & Winston, Inc., 1966.

————. *Kinesics and Context.* Philadelphia: University of Pennsylvania, 1970.

CALVEY, ROSEANN. "Identification of Encouraging and Inhibiting Nonverbal Behaviors of Nurses in Selected Nurse-Patient Interactions and Nonverbal Behaviors Stated by Patients." Unpublished Dissertation, Catholic University, 1972, page 27.

CARSON, RACHEL. The *Silent Spring.* Boston: Houghton Mifflin Company, 1962.

CHISHOLM, FRANCIS P. "A New Kind of Comprehension Test," *Journal of Communication,* Fall, 1955.

ECKERT, ALLEN. *The Silent Sky.* Boston: Little, Brown and Company, 1965.

FERREIRA, N. J. "On Silence," *American Journal of Psychotherapy,* January, 1964.

FRANK, LAWRENCE K. "Tactile Communication," *ETC: A Review of General Semantics,* Vol. 16, Autumn, 1958.

GALLOWAY, CHAS. M. "Nonverbal: The Language of Sensitivity," *Theory Into Practice,* Vol. X, No. 4, October, 1971.

GIBSON, JAMES. "Observation on Active Touch," *Psychological Review,* Vol. 69, November, 1962.

HALL, EDWARD T. *The Silent Language.* Greenwich: Fawcett Publications, Inc., 1959.

————. *The Hidden Dimension.* New York: Doubleday & Company, Inc., 1966.

HALL, EDWARD T., and WHYTE, WM. F. "Intercultural Communication: A Guide to Men of Action," *Human Organization,* Vol. 19, Spring, 1960.

HARTE, THOMAS J., and FURFEY, PAUL H., DOUGLAS, A. M., et al. "Meeting the Health Needs of the Totally Deaf," unpublished report, Department of Social Research, The Catholic University of America, Washington, D. C., 1964.

HAYAKAWA, S. I. "How to Attend a Conference," *ETC: A Review of General Semantics,* Autumn, 1955.

————. *Language in Thought and Action.* New York: Harcourt, Brace and World, Inc., 1949.

HOEBEL, E. ADAMSON. *Man in the Primitive World.* New York: McGraw-Hill Book Company, 1958.

JACOB, STANLEY W., and C. A. FRANCONE. *Structure and Function in Man.* Philadelphia: W. B. Saunders Company, 1965.

KNAPP, MARK L. "The Role of Nonverbal Communication in the Classroom," *Theory Into Practice,* Vol. X, No. 4, October, 1971.

MANOCK, HELEN. "Silence," *Perspectives in Psychiatric Care,* Vol. 2, 1964.

MANSFIELD, ELAINE C. "Role Model Demonstration of Empathic Behaviors With Schizophrenic Patients in Video Taped Nurse-Patient Interviews." Unpublished Doctoral Dissertation, Catholic University, School of Nursing, 1972.

MEERLOO, J. A. M. *Conversation and Communication.* New York: International Universities Press, 1952.

————. "Greeting as a Trial Approval," *Archives of General Psychiatry,* Vol. 15, September, 1966.

MERCER, LIANNE S. "Touch: Comfort or Threat?" *Perspectives in Psychiatric Care,* Vol. 4, 1966.

MONTAGU, ASHLEY. *Touching*. New York: Columbia University Press, 1971.

MORSE, WM. C., and WINGO, G. M. *Psychology and Teaching*. New York: Scott, Foresman and Company, 1955.

ORLANDO, IDA JEAN. *The Dynamic Nurse-Patient Relationship*. New York: G. P. Putnam's Sons, 1961.

POTTER, SIMEON. "Language and Society," Patrick and Mary Hazard (eds.), *Language and Literacy Today*. Chicago: Science Research Associates, Inc., 1965.

RUESCH, JURGEN, and KEES, W. *Nonverbal Communication*. Los Angeles: University of California Press, 1956.

SECORD, PAUL F. "Facial Features and Inference Processes in Interpersonal Perception," *Person Perception and Interpersonal Behavior*, R. Tagiuri and L. Petrullo (eds.). Stanford: Stanford University Press, 1958.

Webster's New World Dictionary. New York: The World Publishing Company, 1957.

ZOLA, IRVING K. "Roundup of Current Research," *Trans-action*, April, 1967.

Perceptions and Feelings

It is impossible to understand communication without an understanding of perception. The field of study, however, is so broad in scope that only a fraction of the knowledge accumulated can be dealt with here.

How we humans perceive the world around us is a continuing concern of psychologists, teachers, psychiatrists, physiologists, and philosophers. A great deal of experimental work has been done in an attempt to identify various factors which influence perception, but much confusion and disagreement continue to exist among various scientists. Numerous studies of perception have led to the development of new learning theories, the study of psychometrics and even semantics, as well as problem-solving techniques and theories regarding attitude change.

Some attention has been centered on studies of "internal" perception as distinct from "external" perception. Russell Mason defines "internal" perception as sensory experiences arising from within the body. During a state of fatigue, for example, a person's cognitive activity is at a minimum, and Mason believes that the person is more aware of bodily sensations and less aware of external sensations. Mason shows that "internal" perception can be differentiated from other kinds of inner experiences such as feeling and emotion—the nature of which is not clearly understood.[1] Most of the studies, however, have focused on the immediate recognition and discrimination of external stimuli, including attention and memory as essential aspects of perception.

Daniel Cappon of Toronto, Canada, has written of the relations and interactions of technology and perception. He discusses the point that

---

[1] Russell E. Mason, *Internal Perception and Bodily Functioning* (New York: International Universities Press, Inc., 1961), pp. 11-36.

technological products change the culture, primarily because they change the modes of perception. Man is changed in thought and in deed by the tools he has made, and the point of impact bringing about change seems to occur "at the level of the senses and percepts of orientation."[2] He too views perception as a process and as one of the mental processes determining behavior. Cappon notes that the primary function of all perception is the recognition of change, with the ultimate aim of adaptation and mastery of the environment.[3] His main thrust is his desire to present the need for and a beginning plan for the development of a perceptual typology. For those interested in perception, his elucidation of some of the complexities of the process of perception will find his writing extremely helpful for study and research.

DEFINITION OF PERCEPTION

Generally, perception is conceived of as the process of becoming aware through our senses. Morse and Wingo give a clear and comprehensive explanation of how we perceive:

> The perception of a given scene is a complex set of reactions including sensory stimulation, organizing forces within the nervous system, symbolic recollections of past experiences, and the arousal of affective responses.[4]

This explanation conveys the fact that human perception includes more than our senses of sight, hearing, smell, taste, and touch. We have ideas, values, concepts, meanings, and perceptions of relationships. Most of our conscious awareness, however, is focused on our external environment, which enables us to know the world around us. People who cannot see or hear are deprived of these perceptions, and consequently their perception of the world is altered.

We use our perceptions to communicate with others, but if we are to report our perceptions to others, we must organize them and name them. In order to do this, David Berlo suggests that we must be selective. How we select depends on our cultural background. That is, the ways in which we have been trained to perceive. Berlo says that cultural background is responsible for the fact that we perceive some things and not others. He also feels that it is the major factor in our making judgments. Judgments are based on our prior experiences and

---

[2]Daniel Cappon, *Technology and Perception* (Springfield: Chas. C Thomas Publisher, 1971), p. 14.
[3]*Ibid.*, p. 85.
[4]William C. Morse and G. M. Wingo, *Psychology and Teaching* (New York: Scott Foresman and Company, 1955), p. 462.

values.[5] Other psychologists have indicated that we cannot attend to all perceptions available, and that we often perceive only those things that have meaning, interest, and value for us. We tend to ignore things that we find distasteful.

As nurses we need to know how we come to an impression of another person. Perception of people is a problem in cognition, that is, a process of knowing or perceiving. Since much of our life is spent in interaction with other people it is pertinent to consider our awareness of each other's needs, thoughts, and emotions. Our evaluation of another person rests on our perception of him. In any person-to-person contact we know that the other person also perceives us. Thus, we have a two-person interaction, each perceiving the other and each influencing the other. In nursing, we speak of the nurse-patient relationship as an integral part of the nursing process, a special two-person interaction.

This interaction is a perceptual situation in which there should be, and usually is, an emotional involvement of both patient and nurse. Included in any person perception is a consideration of the person's past experience in his environment and his culture that provided the formation of his attitudes, feelings, and beliefs.

A nurse has a distinct opportunity to increase her perceptual abilities as she must interact with a variety of persons every day. On the other hand, she may find her ability to comprehend human action baffling if she is not aware of the variety of environmental differences of each person. Frequently, we categorize each person habitually from a limited source of knowledge of human variation, which then limits our perception. If our perception of the other person is limited, this alters and diminishes our interaction with him. Our perception allows us to know more completely a particular person. Nurses are sometimes perplexed by patients who do not wish to divulge their intentions. Some persons do not disclose their wishes or attitudes since to do so allows the other person to have more control over them. In addition, the more we disclose our perceptions, the more we open ourselves to positive or negative criticism. Many male patients would be reluctant to verbalize a fear concerning their condition in view of female nurses' negative responses.

Hadley Cantril enlarges on the concept of social perception which is more specifically related to nurse-patient perceptions. Cantril discusses the nature of social perception and states, "It seems clear that any perception is an awareness that emerges as a result of a most complicated weighing process an individual goes through as his mind takes into ac-

[5]David K. Berlo, *The Process of Communication* (New York: Holt, Rinehart & Winston, Inc., 1960), p. 231.

count a whole host of factors or cues."[6] He reminds us that the integration of all these factors is accomplished in a fraction of a second and is, more frequently than not, entirely unconscious. Cantril believes that perception is part and parcel of purposive activity and can only be understood in this context. That is, in all our relationships, it is the purposes or actions of other people that affect the carrying out of our purposes and the possibility of our purposes affecting the carrying out of theirs. In nursing, it is necessary for us to understand patient's purposes. If we do not, as Cantril notes, "we will be unsuccessful in carrying out our purposes to the extent that we are unaware of the purposes of others. . . ."[7]

INTERFERENCES WITH PERCEPTIONS

Combs and Snygg discuss in detail various factors that inhibit our perceptions, particularly those that relate to our needs. They cite as an example the person who strongly desires respect, but who brags so much that he loses the acclaim he seeks. His strong need for respect narrows his perception. Another inhibiting factor is the concentration upon a particular perception to the point where it is difficult to perceive events in a broader perspective. Trying to remember someone's name is an illustration of this. At other times, such as in emergency situations, concentration on one perception is highly advantageous.[8] Combs and Snygg posit that personal threat is probably the most restrictive on our perceptions. Some threats are physical; others are social, including specific people. Another factor that restricts perception occurs when we are required to defend ourselves against attack. The attacks may be aimed at ourselves personally, or at things which are extensions of ourselves. We defend *our* home, *our* hospital, *our* church often as strongly as we would *our*selves, because they are extensions of us.

Combs and Snygg report an interesting experiment, in which subjects were requested to rate themselves and others before and after a stressful situation. The subjects rated themselves and their friends better when under stress than when not under stress.[9] This has significance in the way patients rate nurses and the way nurses rate patients when both are under stress.

---

[6]Hadley Cantril, "The Nature of Social Perception." *Social Perception.* Hans Toch and H. C. Smith (eds.) (Princeton: D. Van Nostrand Co., Inc., 1968), p. 5.

[7]*Ibid.,* p. 9.

[8]Arthur W. Combs and Donald Snygg, *Individual Behavior* (New York: Harper & Row, Publishers, 1949), pp. 167-168.

[9]*Ibid.,* pp. 172-173.

PERCEPTION AND COMMUNICATION

According to Arthur Combs' view, the behavior of a person is the direct result of his field of perceptions at the moment of his behaving. The three basic principles of this concept are: (1) how the individual sees himself; (2) how he sees the situations in which he is involved; and (3) the interrelations of these two.[10] In order for you to communicate effectively with a patient, it is necessary for you to understand the meaning derived from the first two principles and discover the relations between them. That is, you need to acquire an understanding of the other person's perceptual field before you can communicate effectively with him. Without this information from the other person about his own perceptions, we must work blindly and only from our own perceptions, which are rarely useful to the other person.

The following example reveals this discrepancy: A nurse said to Mr. W_____, "It seems to me, you are not cooperating—you interrupt every one when they speak, and try to be funny about everything." The patient replied, "No one listens when I get serious, and everyone laughs and listens when I joke—I've decided that's the only way I get heard." Not all patients would be this frank, but fortunately this man was able to verbalize his perceptions. In this example the patient was able to perceive himself and the situation in which he was involved. On the other hand, the nurse's comment reflected only her own perception of the situation.

Patients and nurses share different perceptual and cultural worlds. It takes some time for patients to learn the expectations, values, beliefs, and ways of behaving in our hospitals. Whether they should be required to learn this is an important question. Their perceptions of their situations are different than our perception of their situations. We are frequently not aware of their perceptions, and we often imply that they should be aware of ours. Our communication with each other suffers when this occurs.

Human perception is very complex and though there are many theories about how we perceive, many of them are by necessity complex and too detailed for our specific use. It is very difficult to study how another person reacts to stimuli. Generally, we observe the person and make inferences from his reactions, but this procedure has many limitations. We are constantly bombarded by external stimuli and our responses occur automatically within split second timing and are governed

---

[10]Arthur W. Combs, *The Professional Education of Teachers* (Boston: Allyn and Bacon, Inc., 1965), p. 12.

by a multitude of factors. Thus, it is very difficult to make inferences from our observations. The ideas regarding the relation between perception and communication of Combs and Snygg have been presented because they seem to have more practical value for our needs in improving our communication with patients.

THE ROLE OF FEELINGS IN COMMUNICATION

All of us talk rather glibly about our feelings, some feelings relate to our body, some to our emotions, others to things, events, or happenings. We, in our American society, do not generally condone an overt expression of our feelings about other people, or about ourselves. We are taught from early childhood that we don't tell our mother that she doesn't bake as good a cake as Aunt Mary even though Mother's cake doesn't taste as good. We are not allowed to tell Aunt Mary that her nose looks funny, even though we perceive that her nose is an odd shape compared to the shape of the noses of other family members. Girls soon learn that the expression of their feelings about a schoolmate to a close friend is called "gossiping." Children are also taught not to express their true feelings about certain customs established in our society. If a child receives a birthday gift which he doesn't like, he learns that it is not polite to say he doesn't like it—in fact, he is expected to convey to the gift bearer the exact opposite of his feelings—and say that he likes it. In the Middle East, the Arab is permitted, even encouraged, to express his feelings without inhibition. Grown men can weep, shout, gesture expressively and violently, jump up and down—and be admired as sincere.[11] Thus, variations occur in different cultures.

On the other hand, children in our society are allowed to express positive feelings about another person a little more freely, but within limits. It is acceptable for a young child to say, "I like you, mommy"; however, some mothers display a certain embarrassment if an older child expresses a positive feeling toward them, particularly in the presence of friends. It has become appropriate in our society to comment positively on a friend's dress, other wearing apparel, or material possessions. However, this too has its limits, as you would not wish the other person to think you were not accustomed to such luxuries.

In too many families it is not a practice for parents to compliment or encourage an expression of true feelings—negative or positive. How many of you were encouraged to express your feelings of pride, love, or concern

---

[11]Edward T. Hall and Wm. F. White, "Intercultural Communication: A Guide to Men of Action," *Human Organization*, Vol. 19, Spring, 1960, p. 17.

for your parents, brothers, sisters, or friends? Conversely, were you ever encouraged to express your negative feelings about their behavior, dress, or untoward reactions to various persons, including their reactions to you? Obviously, it would not be useful for us to learn to express negative feelings for the sake of expressing them. Most people try to hide their feelings from others, and in view of how we are taught to do so it is not surprising. How one's positive or negative feelings are expressed is always a component that affects acceptance.

This leads us to examine the purpose of our expression of feelings. You may ask "What is the value in expression of feelings?" We are taught that to say to another person we don't like the unfriendly way he treats us will hurt his feelings and inhibit the relationship between us. However, in any relationship, personal or professional, we experience both positive and negative feelings toward the other person. No relationship can exist without both kinds of feelings being present. If we were taught that it would improve our relationship with the other person to discuss the little irritations about that person's behavior which interfere with our acceptance of them, or vice versa, we could learn to change our behavior and enjoy each other's company more fully. For example, I have a friend who once said, "I am not going to sit by you in the meeting, because your smoking bothers me. I like you, but my eyes are irritated by smoke, and I will see you after the meeting." This is a very forthright statement, and allows me to either change my behavior and sit by her or continue to smoke and sit alone. The most important factor is that I know why she is not sitting next to me. If she had not spoken her true feelings, I could have easily misinterpreted her action. It should be also noted that she was not asking me to change my behavior, nor was she annoyed with me. She merely clarified her feelings.

Many people would not verbalize their feelings this easily for fear that they would hurt the other person's feelings, and that it would be "bad" behavior to do so. As long as we continue to consider any negative expression to another person as bad, we will continue to isolate that person from us, and communication with him will be limited.

The main value in the expression of feelings is to allow the other person to know something about what we are experiencing. If I know something about the personal meaning of an event for another person, my communication with that person will be altered. If we were taught also that our feelings are a true representation of our perceptions, then the expression of them would assist us in our relationship with another person, we would not grow up hiding our feelings, and we would be able to alter our behavior to improve our relationships. If we learned that to express our feelings in an angry manner would not improve our relationship, and would perhaps negate communication with that person, we would develop ways to express our feelings in an acceptable manner.

Since people do not easily verbalize their feelings, it is generally unproductive for the nurse to ask, "Tell me how you feel about. . . ." or "Tell me what your feelings are about that." The patient may wonder why the nurse wants to know, or what will her reaction be if he tells her his true feelings, or he would be embarrassed for her to know. Often times it is helpful if the nurse expresses her feelings about a situation, which allows the patient to know that her reaction may not be too different than his own. This allows the patient to more freely express his feelings.

Combs and Snygg believe that feelings are not the cause of our behavior. If you are angry at someone and "tell them off," it is *not* the feeling of anger that causes you to verbalize in this manner, but your perception of the interaction that occurred.[12]

If we were taught that it is safe or acceptable to express positive feelings to another person about their attributes, we would have many more friends. Positive phrases such as "My, you look pretty in that dress," are not only a compliment, but also an indication that the person who makes the statement likes the other person, and indirectly tells them through the comment about their dress. If we were taught to say, "You are a wonderful friend," or "You have a real skill in conveying your thoughts and making another person feel comfortable," our relationship with others would be much more positive.

It is true that some people in our society have been taught how to express both positive and negative feelings toward another person in such a manner that communication is enhanced, but these are the rare individuals. They are so rare, in fact, that we tend to comment on this quality when describing such individuals.

It is one of the ironies of our society that we commonly greet another person with "How are you feeling?" In essence, however, we do not expect a response about feelings. The intent of the message is only to greet the other person—not to inquire about his true feelings. Usually the response is "fine," which may hide the true feelings. Occasionally, someone takes the greeting literally and tells the inquirer how he feels physically and mentally, usually to the surprise of the initiator of the statement. Nurses, unfortunately, are bearers of the same message, and though they may need to know how the patient is feeling, they, too, are often only greeting the patient and do not expect a true answer.

---

[12]Combs and Snygg, *op. cit.*, p. 234.

Most of us are aware that our feelings impede or facilitate our communication, and it is safe to say that we never communicate without expressing our feelings about what we are saying. But what are feelings? "Feelings are a kind of shorthand description of our perceptual fields at a particular moment."[13] Feeling is the symbol we use to describe our awareness of our condition of being, such as, "I feel frustrated." It is, however, difficult to convey to another person just what the feeling is that is being experienced, since no two people are frustrated in exactly the same manner. The same is true for any of the emotions that a person experiences: love, anger, joy, sadness, etc. The manner or the situation that produced the feeling of frustration is never the same for any two individuals.

There are so many differences in our feelings toward our multiple experiences, that it is very difficult to convey to others their subtle or complex meanings. A friend recently remarked, "I feel devastated," which was made in a tone of voice akin to sadness or despair. The subtleness in meaning may need an analogy to assist the listener to gain the true meaning. In order to understand the other person's feeling and offer comfort we would need to recognize that this person has been involved in a situation with one or more persons, and that the nature of this interaction produced the feeling of devastation. Even if we ourselves have experienced devastation, we cannot fully understand what the feeling of devastation means for this person, because each individual is different, and another's interpersonal situation is different from our own. This is one of the difficulties encountered when we attempt to show empathy for another person. No one experiences sadness, love, or anger in exactly the same manner. We can approximate to a degree, but each experience is unique for the individual person.

It is crucial for a nurse to understand that feelings about one's own self can predominate to such an extent that they obscure more appropriate kinds of feelings. If a person experiences an interaction that produces a feeling of devastation, it is highly unlikely that he will be able to experience positive feelings about any segment of his life for a period of time. For some people, this may only be momentary; for others, it may be several weeks, or even longer. Only as he reviews the problem verbally with another individual can he begin to evaluate the interaction which produced the feeling. To understand the development of feelings of this nature, we need to explore further the meaning of feelings.

Feelings relate to an individual's self, that is, the way an individual views himself. Feelings about self influence the way he will react to any

---

[13]*Ibid.,* p. 232.

situation. If a person feels he is worthwhile, self-confident, and compe-
tent, he will more likely experience these feelings when interacting with
others. Even in situations where he is exposed to personal criticism, he
will be more easily able to evaluate the criticism and decide if the evidence is accurate. He will not immediately feel inadequate because of
the criticism, and will attempt to determine the reason for the censure.
He may be startled by the criticism, depending upon the relationship
with the other person. If he knows the critic quite well, he will probably find it easier to be more verbally direct in his inquiry to his friend,
and may be inclined to think of it as a misunderstanding. If he does not
know the person intimately, he may be more cautious in his approach,
but he will still not accept the criticism without inquiry, because he
feels that as a person, he knows no reason for the criticism, and is confident of his self-worth as a person.

Conversely, the person who does not feel self-confident tends to incorporate personal criticism, and frequently is unable to investigate any
criticism. He tends to accept criticism as somehow legitimate. This further lowers his feeling of adequacy as a person. This person may not be
able to verbally inquire about the criticism for fear that the remarks are
true or that his feelings of inadequacy will become evident. He may
experience feelings of anger as a result of this threat to his self-esteem
and be unable to communicate, or he may angrily defend himself as
though the admonition were true. Most persons have a reaction to criticism, but the person who is self-confident is not likely to accept criticism
without first ascertaining the reason for it.

For both the person with high or low self-esteem, criticism produces
feelings which influence their communication, but in different ways. Our
feelings will influence the response we make to someone we like or dislike. A teacher once responded in the following manner to the remark,
"Are we having a meeting today?" made by two different persons, one
whom she liked, the other whom she disliked. "Yes, at two p.m.," was
the response to one person, and to the other the response was, "I suppose
so, we usually do." No explanation is needed to identify which person
was liked.

There has been a trend in the past few years to believe that we should
learn to express our angry feelings. A few words about this overgeneral-
ization seem in order.

At the beginning of this chapter we noted that children are often
taught not to say exactly how they feel. We mentioned that this may impede communication later in life. We need to recognize that there will
usually be a reaction by the person to whom the angry feelings are expressed. It takes great skill to express the *feeling* of anger in a socially

acceptable way. If one stamps one's foot, screams, and uses words which are annihilating in character, the behavior may impart the message, with the words only adding to the intensity of the message. This type of verbal expression of anger is not productive for improving a relationship, and may, in fact, sever it completely. It is not enough to learn to express angry feelings, we must learn how to verbally express the feeling of anger in a manner which the other person can hear.

If we are to understand the role that feelings have in our everyday communication, we, as nurses, need to be knowledgeable about our own ability to express feelings, and our ability to perceive the verbal communications of others' feelings.

BIBLIOGRAPHY

BERLO, DAVID K. *The Process of Communication*. New York: Holt, Rinehart & Winston, 1960.

CANTRIL, HADLEY. "The Nature of Social Perception," *Social Perception*. H. Toch and H. C. Smith, (eds.). Princeton: D. Van Nostrand Company, Inc., 1968.

CAPPON, DANIEL. *Technology and Perception*. Springfield: Chas. C Thomas Publisher, 1971.

COMBS, ARTHUR W. *The Professional Education of Teachers*. Boston: Allyn and Bacon, Inc., 1965.

COMBS, ARTHUR W., and SNYGG, D. *Individual Behavior*. New York: Harper & Row, Publishers, 1949.

HALL, EDWARD T., and WHYTE, WM. F. "Intercultural Communication: A Guide to Men of Action," *Human Organization*, Vol. 19, Spring, 1960.

MASON, RUSSELL E. *Internal Perception and Bodily Functioning*. New York: International Universities Press, Inc., 1961.

MORSE, WM. C., and WINGO, G. M. *Psychology and Teaching*. New York: Scott, Foresman and Company, 1955.

Components of
Nurse-Patient Communication

For some time now, I have been concerned that when we in nursing have discussed communication, we have been focusing too narrowly on interviewing skills. We have implied, perhaps without realizing it, that our communications with patients are totally confined within the framework of an interview. Some nursing authors have used the term "interview" to include all verbal interactions with a patient. Some schools of nursing actually teach the student to spend a specific period of time interviewing the patient. The amount of time considered adequate for this varies from fifteen minutes to an hour. It seems, though this is not always clear, that the sole purpose of the interview is to obtain certain information from the patient; how the information is to be used, or what kind of information sought is also not clear.

Other authors are more explicit and state that the interview refers to a specialized pattern of verbal interaction, initiated for a specific purpose and focused on some specific content area, with consequent elimination of extraneous material. If we adhere to the definition of the word "interview" we find that it means: (1) a meeting face-to-face, a private conversation, a formal meeting for consultation; (2) question or converse with, especially in order to obtain information or ascertain personal qualities.[1]

In the nurse-patient relationship we do meet with the person face-to-face, but most nurses would agree that communicating with the patient is more than just a private conversation. In some instances it may be a meeting which is specifically for consultation purposes. The second area

---

[1]*Webster's New World Dictionary* (New York: The World Publishing Company, 1957), p. 765.

of the definition pertains to obtaining information. If this is what we mean by communicating with patients, I would question our purpose. There may be instances when we do need to obtain certain information from the patient, but this surely should not be our main purpose.

It is true that dictionary definitions are a record of what words have meant to various people in the past. However, they are a guide to interpretation for people who want to know the prevailing usage of a word. We cannot have a word mean anything we wish if we are to have successful communication. We must correctly relate our words to the things or events for which they stand. However, I wish to make it clear that I am less concerned about the definition and more concerned about the meaning or purpose of interviewing.

This section of the book pertains to common uses of language that serve a practical function in communication. These are presented in the hope that they will help you to grasp what the other person is saying. In addition, these uses may help you in communicating more effectively with patients and other people as well.

COMMUNICATION OF TRUST

How does a person communicate trust? How do we let another person know we trust them? How do they let us know we are trusted? In order to answer these questions we must be certain what we mean by trust. The following statement sums up the essence of trust; *when you rely on someone without question, that is trust.* Most of us have a few close friends or relatives with whom we experience trust; some people do not have any one person that they can rely on without question, though this is what all persons strive for in their relationships. In nursing, we often assume that the patient trusts us but we are often faced with mistrust. It is more difficult for us to recognize that we do not foster trust either by our actions or by our communication. We frequently state that we do not trust Mrs. So-and-so, therefore indicating that some behavior of the person leads to mistrust.

Don Jackson notes that the word "trust" originally came from the Scandinavian language and meant "to comfort," "to console," "to confide in." It first appeared in approximately the ninth or tenth century in which men and women lived in a state of relative equality, in an environment requiring a desperate struggle for survival. It then meant to give comfort and cheer when needed, and had nothing to do with estimating another's behavior.[2] The modern meaning of "trust" is quite dif-

---

[2]D. D. Jackson and W. J. Lederer, *The Mirages of Marriage* (New York: W. W. Norton & Company, Inc., 1968), p. 107.

ferent from its original connotation. Today, the meaning of trust encompasses consistency in a person's behavior, including what he verbalizes, though we have learned that one's verbal communication may not be consistent with one's behavior.

Erik Erikson, in describing the development of trust in the infant, includes the need to learn to trust oneself: the general state of trust implies not only that one has learned to rely on the sameness and continuity of others, but also that one must trust oneself.[3] Trust is learned early in life—in infancy. Erikson places trust in the first stage of an infant's development and makes the point that the amount of trust "does not seem to depend on absolute quantities of food or demonstrations of love, but rather on the quality of the maternal relationship.[4] This point is important for nurses in their approach to patients—"It is not how much we give, but the quality of giving." Our ability to trust is learned from our experiences with others, and it is closely associated with our identity. Erikson defines trust as an attitude toward oneself and the world derived from the experiences of the first year of life. It is taught by mothers but in different ways to fit the cultural version of the universe.

Erikson makes it clear that we must also learn mistrust, that is, there must be a certain ratio of trust and mistrust, because "we must be able to differentiate how much we can trust and how much we must mistrust." He uses mistrust "in the sense of a readiness for danger and an anticipation of discomfort."[5]

Thus, it is necessary for the nurse to recognize that the patient must assess the situation and the nurse before he can trust her. The patient who is not aware of a particular treatment may be leery of danger or discomfort until the nurse communicates what to expect or gives information about the treatment.

Concomitant with the development of trust in the child is the development of hope, and, according to Erikson, "is a very basic human strength," which he labels "a virtue." He views hope "as the basic ingredient of all strength, that is, something vital, that animates and is the soul of something." Erikson says, "If life is to be sustained hope must remain, even where confidence is wounded, trust impaired. Hope relies on its beginnings on the new being's first encounter with *trustworthy maternal persons. . . .*"[6] But Erikson also notes that nothing in

---

[3]Erik Erikson, *Childhood and Society*, (2d ed.) (New York: W. W. Norton & Company, Inc., 1950), p. 248.

[4]*Ibid.*, p. 249.

[5]E. E. Evans, *Dialogue with Erik Erikson* (New York: Harper & Row, Publishers, 1967), p. 15.

[6]Erik Erikson, *Insight and Responsibility* (New York: W. W. Norton & Company, Inc., 1964), pp. 115-116.

human life "is secured in its origin unless it is verified in the intimate meeting of partners in favorable social settings." Erikson does not see hope as a static state, but one that has to be confirmed and reaffirmed through life.[7] We all know that we can be very trusting of an individual, but something can be done or said by the person that can alter that trust. It is only through communication that we can clarify the meaning of what the person said or did to reaffirm our trust.

It is through communication that trust can be developed with another person. Communication must be clear and honest. If deception is practiced, trust cannot be established. It is not possible to hide deception, it will leak out eventually. Honesty involves not simply saying what one believes, but also doing what one says. If the nurse says "I want to help you," but never comes to the room to see if the patient needs help, the patient will not believe the nurse. If the nurse tells the patient she will return at nine o'clock but doesn't arrive until 9:15, she invites mistrust, particularly if she does not explain her reason for being late.

Persons who have not learned to trust others easily from past experiences will present even more of a challenge to the nurse. These people tend to mistrust more readily and only through honest communication will they be able to trust the nurse.

It must be remembered that trust is not developed alone, it can only *NB* exist between two people.

If people, for our purposes, the nurse and the patient, can be truthful and open about themselves, mutual support and helpfulness are possible. A generosity in relation to the other person's mistakes becomes easier when we learn that others can be generous in return. If a person can be honest enough to recognize and admit his own weaknesses, he will be forgiven by others and it then becomes possible for him to be tolerant of the weaknesses of others. If we are able to give to people we trust because we have received from them, then it follows that trust and generosity are both causes and results of a genuine give and take. If the nurse is able to state to the patient that she honestly forgot to bring him his medication, the patient is more likely to be tolerant of her lapse of memory. Likewise, the nurse must be able to be tolerant of the patient's lapse of memory, as when he forgets to save a urine specimen. In both these instances there must be an honest communication about the memory loss. If the nurse had to cover up and say "Oh I thought someone else had given it," when she knew she had forgotten, this is deceptive. When the nurse is able to be honest, the patient knows he can trust her. Likewise, if the patient says, "I didn't know I was supposed to save a

---

[7]Evans, *op. cit.*, pp. 17-18.

specimen," when in fact he did know but did not wish to be thought forgetful, this too is deceptive. Trust is possible when verbal and nonverbal behavior are consistent and are communicated clearly. It is very difficult to lie to someone and not give out nonverbal clues that are inconsistent to the verbal communication. Even though in our society there is a taboo against lying, it is a rare person who does not at some time or other lie about something. Lying or deceit is the basis of mistrust, as honesty is the basis of trust. We generally are not honest when we feel we have failed or are not "perfect." Being human includes possessing frailities and it takes a great deal of courage to honestly communicate. Yet the rewards are greater for establishing trust. Trust requires constant exercise of intelligence, truthfulness, and courage. Perhaps that is why it is so rare.

A basic requirement for trusting another person is related to one's self-esteem or identity, as mentioned earlier. If we do not see ourselves as worth while and do not trust our own actions, it is impossible to trust others. If one is afraid to be honest in his communications about his own feelings and ideas, that is, he is not certain they are valid or he is afraid of repercussions, then the person cannot be honest or trust his own actions.

In summary, if a nurse expects a patient to trust her, she must be aware that her actions and communications will be the deciding factors which will or will not allow the patient to rely on her without question.

INFORMATION (GIVING AND RECEIVING)

Earlier, it was stated that the amount of information we receive through our senses is remarkable. How much information we receive verbally would be difficult to determine, but it is probably quite meager in comparison to the total input of sensory information. Generally, people are often hesitant to inform others about themselves and their activities until they are acquainted with the other person. Even at the acquaintance stage, some people hesitate to share personal information. There is always the question of how the other person will receive personal information, and this fear can often be a deterrent to the free flow of personal information from one person to another.

In nursing, there are instances when it is necessary and vital that we have specific information from patients in order to assist them. We need to know when they are in physical pain or mental anguish. We may need information about their diet, their sleep patterns, their elimination, and their fears, as well as many other personal things. As nurses, we have little need for information about the number of children a patient has, or about his marital state, age, number of hospitalizations, religion, occupation, location of residence, social values, and income. Except for religion, (in time of death) and occupation (if it interferes with health), we could give excellent nursing care without any knowledge of these other social characteristics. Unfortunately, information is sought more frequently about these items than the physical and psychological ones.

The social items are usually obtained by a clerk for the record, and become a part of the health and illness statistics of a given community or hospital. This is the main reason for obtaining this type of information. It is crucial that we consider the reasons why we, as nurses, wish this information, because it is what we might do with it that troubles the patients. This is highly personal information, and though you may believe it is as important as the physical and psychological information, the difference is that the patient comes to us for assistance with a problem in either the physical or psychological area—he does not come to us to be assisted with his personal status in society!

Because we are human, we allow our bias about divorce, illegitimacy, religion, and social values to influence our attitudes, which in turn influence our nursing care of patients, particularly those who do not fit our stereotype of proper social and moral values. It is not uncommon to hear nurses remark, "That's the Jewish man in Room 16," or "Mrs. Gotrocks is in again," and "That lawyer knows all the answers." Sometimes we even refer to the person by their disease—"The colostomy in Room 211," or "the heart case." In either situation we use the personal information about the person, not as a means of improving our communication but in a manner that implies judgments against the person.

We often proceed in the same way with psychiatric patients who are frequently less able to cope with our verbal demands for information. Not long ago, a middle-aged woman in a mental hospital came to me and said, "Why does that student nurse want so much information about my past life? I have told her everything I can think of, but each week she comes again. What does she do with this information?" Since this was not my student, I could not give her an answer. I doubt that the student nurse knew what she wanted the information for either!

It is very important that nurses learn to communicate with patients in such a way that they obtain the information they need to assist the patient with his health problems. If we cannot deal with certain information we receive, perhaps we would give better nursing care without it.

What seems more important in nurse-patient communication is the kind of information that patients *need* from nurses. Nursing literature abounds with various lists and reminders regarding the kind of information a person needs when entering a hospital. Most of it relates to the physical environment and expectations regarding the "patient role." Much of this information is helpful to the patient, particularly if it is in written form, so that he can refer to it when needed, after his initial anxiety has subsided. It is inevitable that in this new world—the medical or psychiatric sanctuary—he will be faced with a barrage of words which are new symbols with which he is not familiar. All sorts of new activities surround him that are completely foreign in nature. He finds that he really doesn't understand half of the words spoken, most of which are said "on the run" by someone who he hopes is a nurse. In a psychiatric hospital he may even find that everyone is in civilian clothes. Who is the nurse? The old signs are no longer available. To confound the communication problem, the nurse announces that he is to have a CBC and an EKG. Now, letters become substituted symbols for words. Someone asks if he would like some "nourishment." He accepts, only to discover that "nourishment" consists of a cold drink. The "coffee, tea, or milk" airline message is at least understandable, though limited in choice.

The psychiatric patient learns that he is scheduled for the TAT and the Rorschach. Is the latter a kind of "shock"? Language *is* the fundamental mechanism of human survival! Unfortunately, the ordinary types of verbal information patients need so badly is too often withheld from them by inadequate communication.

What other kinds of information do patients require? Some of it is made explicit by the patient, and some must be ascertained through nonverbal signs. The myriad kinds of information a patient needs about his physical or psychological state of health are very difficult to enumerate. They are difficult because they are highly individual in nature. They could relate to physical safety, self-respect, independence, understanding, or general cognitive needs, or any of the gamut of human needs. Some patients will be able to directly ask for information related to their needs; others may be unable to do so, and it will be necessary to be alert to nonverbal cues.

I am reminded of a young man who had been receiving intravenous glucose for a number of weeks. Because of cardiac impairment, the glucose was administered slowly (10 gtts. per minute). As the cardiac impairment improved, the drops per minute were increased. The patient was found pressing the tubing against the bed cradle to lessen the drops. He was scolded for this behavior, and threatened with hypodermoclysis if he did not desist. To his good fortune, a student nurse informed him that his cardiac condition had improved and that the physician had ordered the increased rate of fluid flow. The patient verbally expressed relief and no longer attempted to regulate the flow of fluid. An entire treatment procedure could have been altered, at the expense of discomfort to the patient, had the information not been provided. One can only wonder why the physical improvement was not communicated to the patient. Who doesn't want to know that they are better? In this instance the patient was being blamed for his behavior, when in reality his behavior was due to lack of communication by staff.

On the other hand, many nurses are alert and take note of their patients' many needs. One young nurse, after listening to an angry patient describe a situation involving several patients for whom he voiced concern, responded, "You have great feeling for others, this must be why other patients rely on you." The information that the student provided the patient about his positive feelings for others was exceedingly helpful, since the patient had previously been focusing solely on his limitations.

A great number of illustrations could be given, but these two examples indicate how various kinds of information can be required, and pinpoint the difficulty in making explicit the exact kind of information that patients need about themselves. It is helpful to know the general categories of physical and psychological needs of all humans. With this basic knowledge, the nurse must then endeavor to ascertain, through verbal as well as nonverbal channels, the kinds of information each patient requires. This is an important communication function of the care-giving role.

Understanding

Previously, in discussing successful communication, it was noted that we need to accept the other person's point of view, how he perceives, and how he feels. If we are able to do this, understanding occurs and communication is possible.

Carl Rogers hypothesized that one major barrier to mutual interpersonal communication is "our very natural tendency to judge, to evaluate, to approve or disapprove, the statement of the other person, or the other group."[8] For example, you go to a nurses' meeting or read a book and say, "I didn't like that nurse's talk or that author." Your response will invariably be either approval or disapproval of the attitude expressed. You may respond, "I didn't either. I thought it was terrible," or you reply, "Oh, I thought it was really good." In essence, you have just evaluated what has been said to you from your point of view.

Or in another example, said with feeling, "I think the A.N.A. is really helping nurses get better jobs and higher pay." The likelihood is that you will begin to evaluate the statement and agree or disagree or make some judgment about the speaker such as, "She must not like the NLN,"

---

[8]Carl Rogers, *On Becoming a Person* (Boston: Houghton Mifflin Company, 1961), p. 330.

or "All ANA'ers only think about salaries," or "She's loyal and is an asset to the profession."

Rogers notes that "Although the tendency to make evaluations is common in almost all interchange of language, it is very much heightened in those situations where feelings and emotions are deeply involved. So the stronger our feelings, the more likely it is that there will be no mutual element in the communication. There will be just two ideas, two feelings, two judgments, missing each other in psychological space."[9] Rogers believes that forming an evaluation of the other person's statement is one of the major barriers to interpersonal communication.

How can we overcome this to reach an understanding? To do so takes courage and developing a new approach. It means: I must try and understand how the situation appears to him. I must attempt to solve a problem, not attack the person for his views. Carl Rogers suggests an experiment which he found useful in promoting understanding. He suggests that the next time you find yourself in an argument with your friend, husband, patient or teacher, stop the discussion and follow this approach. "Each person can speak up for himself only *after* he has first restated the ideas and feelings of the previous speaker's accurately, and to that speaker's satisfaction."[10] In other words, before you offer *your* rebuttal, it would be necessary for you to really understand his thoughts and feelings so you could summarize them. It will not be easy. You will find that your own comments will have to be revised, but emotion will be lessened and differences will be reduced. This approach is not the same as reflection. Reflection is only a repetition of the words of the speaker and does not attempt to get at the other person's meaning by restatement. The need to restate in your own words is necessary, because words are not what they seem—the meaning is in the person. This point may seem to be repetitious as it has been stated in various ways throughout this book, but the reemphasis is necessary because of its importance for mutual communication.

Each of us could recall many examples of communication that did not foster understanding. The following instances may assist you in achieving understanding.

(a) Suppose it is one of those mornings when everything on the Unit seems to go wrong. The telephone rings, the nursing assistant is in tears, and you have just spilled a medication on the floor. The supervisor arrives and says, "Why is everything in such a mess here today? Can't you learn to control the situation?" Imagine your response! Suppose, however, the supervisor said, "Mercy,

---

[9]*Ibid.*, p. 331.
[10]*Ibid.*, p. 332.

Miss＿＿＿＿＿ this must be a rough morning for you—how can I help?" The difference in the latter response is that the supervisor didn't attack or criticize you, she understood you, and did not blame you or tell you how to improve.

(b) A patient puts on her light and a nurse comes to the room and asks, "May I help you?" The patient responds, "Yes, I haven't had my twelve o'clock medication. I'm just not getting the care here that I should have." The nurse responds, "I'm terribly sorry, I will get your medication. Is there any other care you wish?" Patient, "No, it's just that my doctor said it was very important that I take the medicine on time." The nurse responds, "I can understand your concern. It is an important medicine and you should have it on time." In this instance the nurse accepts the patient's statement and wishes to understand the patient's view of her care.

What if the nurse had responded to the patient's first statement in the following manner: "Now Mrs. X, I'm sure you've had your medication and forgotten, and there's nothing wrong with your care." In this instance the nurse does not accept the patient's statement, evaluates her as being forgetful, and indicates she cannot judge her care. No communication has occurred and the nurse does not understand. The patient will no longer trust the nurse and will doubtless become more anxious about her medication.

(c) The instructor remarks to a new class of nursing students that we, as a faculty, wish to achieve a genuine understanding of their views and their feelings about their program. Several weeks later, Miss X states, "I do not understand why we must study the history of nursing. It doesn't help us to learn how to be nurses—what is past is past." The instructor responds, "We believe that in order to understand the present, in order to see changes and gain an appreciation of the work accomplished by other nurses, one must understand the past. Is that what you're concerned about?" Student, "No, I can understand that, but this semester is so heavy, we cannot appreciate or take the time to consider anything but the present. The instructor responds, "I can understand your concern. Do you think it would be more meaningful and you would have more time later in the program?" Student, "I'm not certain about more time later, but I would hope to feel more confident about my nursing skills and could concentrate more on the history." If the instructor had stopped with her comments about the necessity for the course and had not asked about the student's concern, she would not have been able to understand why the student asked the question and would have evaluated her question only from her own frame of reference.

It must be reiterated that mutual communication can only occur if we learn to try and understand what the other person is trying to tell us. This approach leads to the discovery of truth that will prevent failure of communication, which is so prevalent in our society today. This cannot occur if we first evaluate their communication from our point of view and without clarification or restatement.

CLARIFICATION

If we wish to be fully understood in our daily communication, we must often clarify our remarks. It is necessary to remind ourselves that our words are not things; the meanings are in us. If I say, "She is a nurse," I am speaking about a particular person, and not all nurses. The statement, "She is a good nurse," reflects my meaning about that person; it tells you no more than this. If you inquire about the meaning of "good," you find out more specifically what I mean, and I have clarified. Whether you agree or disagree with their meanings is not the issue. However, confusion may result when we have differences of opinion, if we do not clarify our meaning.

In the past few years, much confusion has resulted from differences of opinion regarding the merits of diploma or baccalaureate education for nurses. Some nursing educators believe that diploma education is adequate and good; others believe that only baccalaureate education is adequate, and is superior. This difference of opinion is what Hayakawa calls "two-valued orientation." Strong feelings of "good" and "bad" are expressed, and many underlying issues are covered up.[11] It generally produces a combative spirit and few results. In order to come to some understanding, additional distinctions regarding each program must be made which will allow for multi-valued orientation. The resulting clarification of issues will assist in adjusting differences, enabling more rational estimates of each form of nursing education.

As with most two-valued misunderstandings, neither side of an argument is all bad or all good. This kind of problem can exist in evaluation of patient care. I once encountered a situation where part of the nursing staff on a given unit said, "This patient is making no progress; he should be transferred." Several other members of the staff countered with the following, "Oh, yes he is. He is nearly ready to go home." By systemati-

---

[11]S. I. Hayakawa, *Language in Thought and Action* (New York: Harcourt, Brace & World, Inc., 1949), pp. 221-235.

cally examining nursing interaction notes, over a period of time, it was found that the patient had numerically less excited episodes; the episodes were less intensive in nature, and the verbalizations were less distorted. There was evidence that significant improvement had occurred, but the episodes had not totally disappeared. With this additional information, the two groups could recognize their over-generalizations and modify their perceptions. It was thus necessary to clarify the actual situation in order to reconcile the differences of opinion.

We can facilitate understanding if we attempt to view the other person realistically from their frame of reference. By this I mean that each of our life experiences differs, and thus our views about life differ. I am continually amazed to find how many people expect others to view things and people according to their own views. We expect patients to behave in ways that *we* think are appropriate. Nursing educators do not want students to deviate from certain expectations. Mothers and fathers wish their children to follow certain standards. All of us have individual differences because of our past experiences, and we all develop different values due to changes in our society. This does not mean that we should condone all behaviors, or accept all individual value systems. It does mean that we must recognize that there are differences in individuals, and that we should attempt to understand the individual through communication. To dismiss, ignore, criticize, or admonish people for their differences in behavior is destructive.

One of the false notions about listening that we in nursing seem to have developed is that patients always mean something else than what they say. Nurses seem to be educated to listen for something "other" than what is said. I think this has been a detriment to effective nurse-patient communication. It is true that for various reasons many people do not clearly state what is on their mind, but we make a definite error when we arbitrarily decide that the person means something other than what he says. Instead, when we are in doubt as to what the patient really means, we should ask for clarification. Statements such as, "Did you mean . . . ?" or "I'm not certain what you meant to ask me," are helpful in gaining clarification.

A great deal of clarification is necessary if we expect to understand other people's views. Sometimes when we have to clarify our own views, we are surprised to learn that we have insufficient evidence for our own beliefs. One requirement that hastens understanding is the belief that the patient, or any other person, can understand. This further requires that we explain in a different way if understanding does not occur on the first try. Many people believe that psychiatric patients cannot understand because they are confused, stupid, disoriented, etc. It has been my experience that if we believe they can, they are more apt to understand. If you think someone can't understand you, you will not present your messages in the same way as when you believe you can be understood. It is again the problem of dismissing a person on the basis of a preconceived idea of his inability to comprehend.

If I taught a group of students who were confused about a certain theory and believed they would never understand it, probably very little would be communicated. If, on the other hand, I believed that with clarification and explanation students could understand, my communication would be different and understanding would be more apt to occur.

Because they think that patients will not understand what they are saying, many physicians and nurses will talk about a patient's condition in his presence. It is true that the medical vocabulary is not the everyday language, but our general population is better educated today, and many medical terms do appear in our daily papers and periodicals. Nurses should be careful not to assume too much about a patient's inability to understand.

FEEDBACK

"The concept of feedback in cybernetics is used to *describe* a self-regulating machine. Such a machine monitors its environment, interprets conditions of the environment, and regulates itself to meet changing situations. . . ." A common example is a thermostat.[12]

The biological and behavioral sciences have borrowed from this concept. In relation to homeostasis, feedback serves as the process by which the human organism can determine the effectiveness of its adjustive responses. The extent to which this process in a human being is mechanical and predictable, in a biological and psychological sense, is yet to be demonstrated.[13] The model is presented here mainly for information and clarification since the term is in frequent use.

We do know, however, that feedback in communication does influence a person's behavior. What you say to me, and how I respond, involves the "action-reaction-interdependence" of the feedback concept. A simplified explanation of the concept is as follows: one individual performs an act (asks a question, or makes a statement). This is perceived by a second individual who responds and reacts to the original message. This reaction is called feedback. The exchange of messages continues from

---

[12]David W. Merrill, "Interpersonal Feedback: Key to Effective Communications," *Proceedings of the 1967 Institute in Technical and Industrial Communications,* Colorado State University, 1967, p. 83.
    [13]*Ibid.*

one person to another, and becomes a circular process. "An initial message affects the response that is made to it; the response affects the subsequent response, etc. Responses affect subsequent responses because they are utilized by communicators as feedback—as information that helps them determine whether they are achieving the desired effect."[14] The following example is an interchange which represents the desired effect of feedback:

Patient: "I cried all last night because the doctor told me I can't go home this weekend."

Nurse: "Are you disappointed?"

Patient: "In a way. I don't mind staying a few more days, but I guess that means I'm not doing so well."

Nurse: "Do you think that's the reason he won't let you go?"

Patient: "What other reason can there be?"

If feedback had not occurred the situation could have resembled the following:

Patient: "I cried all last night because the doctor told me I can't go home this weekend."

Nurse: "Would you like to go for a walk?"

Patient: "Not now."

Nurse: "Why not?"

Patient: "I didn't sleep last night and I'm tired."

In the second situation, the response to the first statement was not related to the question—the desired effect was not achieved. Subsequent responses altered the message, but the final response was one more attempt to return to the initial statement. We could describe these two situations by merely stating that the nurse verbally dealt with the patient's concern in the first instance and avoided doing so in the second. This would tend to focus attention on the nurse, which is not the purpose of this explanation. Many people function consistently in either fashion —nurses are no exception. The main point is that the feedback concept assists in an analysis of communication by providing a structure which can help us to improve our communication. More specifically, it allows us to examine "what has gone wrong" when we didn't get our message across.

One further comment should be made in relation to this structure. It is not the simple stimulus-response model that is often used to describe reflexive behavior. The stimulus-response model does not explain the complexity of human interchange. Many other factors are present in

----

[14]David K. Berlo, *The Process of Communication* (New York: Holt, Rinehart & Winston, Inc., 1960), pp. 111-116.

every verbal exchange which influence how we respond. None of us is immune to these factors, though some influence certain individuals more than others. For example, if you are my boss or my Dean, I will not respond to you in the same way that I would to my peers or an intimate friend. Thus the position of authority influences how we respond to one another. What we have been taught about and what we have learned from authority figures influences how we think we should behave toward them.

How each of us perceives ourselves is one of the most important factors that influences our communication. Do I respect my ideas? Do I believe I am a capable, trustworthy, and sincere individual, or do I pretend I am this kind of person? In other words, our self-esteem influences how we initiate messages with others, as well as how we respond. Some people have difficulty accepting compliments and they tend to brush them aside as though they didn't believe the speaker. Other people cannot accept criticism. Their view of themselves does not incorporate human limitations.

Our social class can become a barrier to or can facilitate communication. Whether we are a member of the jet-set, or the local agricultural association, determines in part our use of language and the messages we exchange. Our economic position, our occupation or profession, race, religion, political views, all comprise cultural influences that alter our views of one another. Along with status and prestige, we develop expectations of each other, based on these factors. The expectations we develop affect our actions towards others. Students at all levels of education soon learn the expectations of a given professor and communicate accordingly if they wish to receive good grades.

The following story illustrates how our expectations influence our views of others. Several years ago a sociologist was visiting families in the poverty areas of Appalachia. While talking to one farmer, he asked him why he did not leave and seek work elsewhere. The farmer replied that he would leave if he could read the road signs. The sociologist had not considered the possibility of illiteracy in his expectations of the farmer.

In the following situation, it is even more evident how expectations limit our communication. An American Indian woman, during her second pregnancy, had been requested by the Public Health Nurse to attend the prenatal clinic. On each of three visits the woman promised the nurse that she would attend the clinic. However, she never went. When asked why she thought this occurred, the nurse responded, "Indians do not like the white man's ways." Exploration of their communication revealed that the nurse had *no* idea why the patient did not go to the clinic, or even if the Indian woman knew the reason for the nurse's request. The nurse's expectations regarding the patient's attitude severely hindered her assistance to the patient.

Thus, it can be seen that various factors such as authority, self-perception, social class, education, and expectations of others can affect our verbal exchanges with one another. Many other factors not included here also influence our responses. It is hoped that the examples presented will assist you in understanding that various factors influence the process of feedback in our daily communication with one another.

QUESTIONS

Questions are an integral part of our daily conversations, though individual variations occur regarding the number, kind, and frequency of their use. The way we question others is a highly individual trait. There are some general purposes of questions, namely: to gather information, to clarify the meaning of a verbal message, and to ascertain another's thinking about a specific topic. Questions of this nature can help us discover where the similarity between our own and another person's understanding begins and ends.

There are many other uses of questions, many of which evoke emotional responses in the recipient. Questions which indicate a curiosity or prying questions of a personal nature are often resented because the recipient does not know the purpose of the inquiry. Similar questions about others fall into the gossip category and can elicit resentment or sheer delight.

Questions may be designed to indicate that one is stupid if the answer is not known. Some persons delight in "needling" interrogation, usually consciously designed to give discomfort to the receiver. Occasionally, questions are asked for what appears to be clarification, but are designed to show how wrong the other person is, and to score a personal victory. Another kind of question is the "you mean you don't even know that?" type, which is meant to emphasize a high degree of stupidity in the recipient, while simultaneously conveying the questioner's intellectual superiority. All forms of questioning which are derogatory to other people are beyond the rules of conversation, and generally produce a negative impression of the questioner—not the recipient.

Other kinds of emotion-producing questions are those which purport to elicit feelings. "Tell me how you feel?" "Do you feel angry?" "Do you want to share your feelings?" When we are asked these kinds of questions, we are often unaware of how the other person will react if we tell them how we feel; particularly if we explain that we are miserable or distraught. Try these kinds of questions on your friends and observe their responses. You may hear, "Why do you want to know?" "What business is it of yours?" or "What can you do, if I tell you?" It is sort of useless to ask someone if they feel angry when nonverbal (or verbal) messages make it quite clear that they are angry.

If a patient states that he feels worried or tense, it is helpful to ask if something has recently occurred or if there is something you can help with. To ask "would you care to talk about it?" is vague, and leaves him to wonder what he should say about "it." The question does not allow for further feedback if his answer should be "no." We must also learn that when we ask questions of patients, we must anticipate the kind of an answer the question will receive. One should anticipate that the answer to the question "Don't you know better than that?" will elicit a totally different response than the question "Hasn't anyone informed you about this?" In other words, it is necessary to learn to phrase our questions in such a way that they will elicit the answers that we need.

Questions of an imperative nature often carry the impact of probing for information and have all the characteristics of an investigation: "Can't you tell me more?" "Don't you want to explain?" "How can you possibly believe that?" "Will you talk about it?" Implied in some of these questions is that no answer will make one vulnerable to suspect. Again, it reflects back on the person asking the question. The implication is that the questioner is trustworthy and that the recipient should feel free to respond.

We as nurses frequently assume that patients should feel no restraint in freely disclosing their innermost thoughts. We should consider what criteria we use to make this assumption. How much time do *you* need before you confide in a stranger? On what basis do you decide *you* can confide in another person?

Interrogative words such as why, what, where, when, how, and who are also imperative in nature. They demand a response: "Where were you?" "When were you born?" "How did you do it?" "What is your income?" "Why did you come to the hospital?" or "Who cares for your children?" Some people feel that these words assist in gaining information. I would agree with this, but it seems to me these words only elicit certain kinds of information, and do not always elicit necessary information. They are generally useful in situations which require specific facts about a person or an incident, or when the person is aware of the reasons for the questions. However, many questions of this type are totally inappropriate: "Why can't you behave like your sister?" "What do you believe is the cause of your trouble?" "How will you help yourself?" "Who will care for you?" These kinds of questions often stimulate "I don't know" answers, or require information that the person doesn't have. It is easy to imply censure toward the person who asks these types of questions, and it is difficult to know what kind of feedback is desired.

Few of us ask questions which offer comfort or assistance. We should ask this type more often: "May I help you?" or in some instances, "Can I help you?" when we are not certain whether it is possible to help the other person. Other questions which offer assistance may include observations of physical or emotional states. "You look very tired," or "You appear to be angry—can I help you in some way?" and "Would you like some help?" are examples of this kind of question.

Particularly for persons engaged in providing service to others, it is necessary to ask these questions, because some people dislike asking for a service even though they are entitled to it. Many teachers and professionals, as well as clerks in department stores, airline agencies, various kinds of offices, and many service workers are increasingly less inclined to offer assistance spontaneously, via the question, "May I help you?" To be able to assist another person is the essence of life. The aim of all communication is to facilitate our relationships with others. If we did not assist others, there would be little meaning to life.

There are times when it is necessary to ask a question in which the meaning may not be clear and would cause the patient to wonder why you ask. You should ask the question and add, "I am asking this question because . . . ," or, "the reason I'm asking this question is . . . ." For example, you might need to know if a patient had recently taken a specific drug, because it could interfere with a test scheduled for him. It does not take much imagination to know that the patient would be quite concerned if you had not added your reason for your question.

Questions are frequently needed for clarification, and are generally helpful in understanding the other person's views. They usually take the following form, "Would you mind restating your point; I'm not certain I understand?" "Did you mean you were for or against . . .?" or "If I understand you correctly, you mean. . . . ?"

All of us have difficulty putting our ideas into clear statements, and sometimes our listeners use words which have a different meaning for us. Thus, it is necessary to clarify. However, this should never seem like criticism, skepticism, or disagreement.

Additional kinds of questions could be presented and categorized in a different manner than those presented here. The intention has been to present some of the common ones that seem to cause problems. It is very necessary to always consider your purpose in asking any question, to decide how to present the question, and to evaluate your results. The response you receive is more dependent on your question than the person to whom it is directed.

We should also remember that questions must be designed for the patient's benefit. The quantity of information is less important than the responses of your patient, and how helpful you have been. Students are sometimes motivated to ask many unnecessary questions because they are required to write interaction notes for the instructor. This need for "something" on paper is often done at the patient's expense. It would be more advantageous for all of us to keep notes on what kinds of questions assist the patient in obtaining what he needs while in our care.

CONSIDERING THE PATIENTS' PERCEPTIONS

Perceptions were discussed in Chapter 4 in relation to their influence on communication. To provide for an operational understanding, additional information is needed in order to carry out the helping role. To reiterate the perceptual view—"In order to understand a person more completely, we must know how he perceives himself, others, and events around him."

Nurses in the past have tended to rely less on the patients' perceptions, and more on their own observations—*nurses'* perceptions. We have accumulated a great deal of knowledge about human behavior, and, in conjunction with other disciplines, we have accepted various meanings for human behavior. Having accepted these meanings as indicative of certain characteristics of human behavior, it became easy to make judgments about the person. Rarely did we validate our impressions with the patient. In other words, we imposed our perceptions on the patient's perceptual world, and did not include his perceptions in the formulation of our judgments. This in turn altered our communication with and about the patient, and often influenced our attitude toward him.

If we are to become effective nurses, we must take into account patients' perceptions. Furthermore, we must examine our own perceptions and learn the effective communicative skills necessary for ascertaining the perceptions of others.

An illustration may assist in clarifying a patient's perceptual view of his environment. A nurse once observed that a patient appeared bored with the admission procedure and "acted as though he knew all about it." From nonverbal cues, the nurse perceived behavior which indicated boredom. Certain actions, though not specified, gave the impression that "he knew all about it." Both of these observations represented her perception of the patient's behavior. A common practice would be for the nurse to accept her own perception as accurate. But what about the patient's perceptions? How could we ascertain whether or not he was bored? One could ask him if he was familiar with the procedure. If the patient's response was in the negative, you would then wonder what other factors could provoke this behavior. It would be feasible to ask if there was something you could do for him, or if there was something specific he would like to know. From this point on, the feedback from the patient would provide additional clues. If the patient's response to your first question had been "yes," your impression would be confirmed. However, you should offer a way of making the procedure more interesting. It would be possible to ascertain if he had previously been a patient, which would not necessitate repeating the procedure or checking to see if the patient had information on new additions. Who wants to hear an admission procedure repeated if one month or six months previously he had heard the same thing?

This may seem tedious, but it takes more time to write about it, than it would take for you to do it. By doing it, you will have learned much more about the patient, ascertained his perceptions, and been much more helpful. In addition, your attitude toward the patient would have been changed—at least it seems reasonable to predict that it would have changed. You would not have made a cursory observation and left him. The patient would have the impression that you were interested in what he thought. In summary, you would have communicated.

It should be clear from the previous discussions that our individual perceptions govern our actions. How we perceive ourselves predisposes our perceptions of others — in other words, our self-concept. What we believe about ourselves affects everything we do, including our communication. In nursing, we have been negligent, and paid too little attention to the patient's self-concept. If we would do so, we would be less critical of patients' behavior and we would alter our communication with them.

It is not possible, nor appropriate here, to discuss in detail the development of self-concept other than to say that it is something each of us learns through our experiences with others. We learn about ourselves from others through verbal and nonverbal communication. If a child is told repeatedly that he is stupid, he will eventually develop the idea that he is stupid even though in reality he may be highly intelligent. Because human beings can change throughout their entire life span, we have an obligation to help patients to view themselves more realistically.

It is possible to gain information about a person's self-concept if we listen to his verbal self-descriptions of what he can or cannot do and how he perceives others and the situations around him. There is always the problem of how accurately we perceive ourselves. We often verbally overstate or understate our perceptions. It should be recognized that you will need a great deal more understanding about self-concept, but it is not possible for our purposes here to go into detail. However, it is possible to recognize that it is through communication with another that we become aware of and develop our own self-concept.

If a patient tells you she cannot turn over in bed without assistance—her perception is that physically she is not able to do so. Let us not say, "You could do it, if you try," but let us help her learn how to do it, and praise her for accomplishing the task. The underachiever in school, who has the intellectual potential, can be helped to learn, if he is convinced that he is not inadequate. Psychiatric patients often say, "I can't talk with people—I don't make any sense." The nurse needs to recognize that the patient's perception of himself, for whatever reasons, is that he is not able to get other people to understand him. The nurse must indicate that he makes sense to her, and attempt to have the patient identify situations in which he felt he was not understood.

Evidence about our self-concept can also be recognized by the judgments we verbalize about others. Rarely does the person recognize consciously that his comments about others reveal his own shortcomings. Statements such as, "She is so disorganized," "He is a flirt," "He thinks he's so great," are often precipitated by our own feelings of inadequacies in these areas. We should not assume this is true, however, until we have the opportunity to observe the person's behavior.

This brief overview of patient's perceptions has been made to show that we can ascertain a patient's perception of self, others, and his environment, through his verbalizations. If we can learn how to become more skillful in our communication, we can avoid relying on cursory observations for determining judgments of patients' behavior, and we will be able to better assist patients and improve our own image as a helping person.

In this chapter an attempt has been made to examine some components of communication that exist in all nurse-patient interactions. These particular components were chosen for examination because they are the ones that seem most fundamental as to whether or not we communicate effectively with patients.

BIBLIOGRAPHY

BERLO, DAVID K. *The Process of Communication.* New York: Holt, Rinehart & Winston, Inc., 1960.

ERIKSON, ERIK. *Childhood and Society.* (2d ed.) New York: W. W. Norton & Company, Inc., 1950.

————. *Insight and Responsibility.* New York: W. W. Norton and Company, 1964.

EVANS, E. E. *Dialogue with Erik Erikson.* New York: Harper & Row, Publishers, 1967.

HAYAKAWA, S. I. *Language in Thought and Action.* New York: Harcourt, Brace & World, Inc., 1949.

JACKSON, DON D., and LEDERER, W. J. *The Mirages of Marriage.* New York: W. W. Norton and Company, 1968.

MERRILL, DAVID W. "Interpersonal Feedback: Key to Effective Communications," Proceedings of the 1967 *Institute in Technical and Industrial Communications,* 1967.

ROGERS, CARL. *On Becoming a Person.* Boston: Houghton Mifflin Company, 1961.

Webster's New World Dictionary. Cleveland: The World Publishing Company, 1957.

Chapter _____ 6

Criteria
for Examining
Patient's Communication

It should now be clear that communication is an integral part of any nurse-patient interaction. We rely on verbal and nonverbal messages between the nurse and the patient to facilitate nursing care. In the future, monitoring systems will doubtless be used to feed us specific physiological information, thereby providing us with more time for communication with patients.

What we need now is a means of examining any person's communication over a period of time (days or months), in order to arrive at some guidelines for a general plan of action. Many factors influence the extent to which we can communicate with patients. Time is one factor over which we have little control. Many patients are hospitalized for short periods of time, and we have little opportunity to get to know them. We frequently have longer contacts with public health and psychiatric patients, the aged, and, in some instances, hospitalized children—including the mentally retarded.

An important dimension of the time factor is how much time you literally spend with the patient. It need not be pointed out that if you converse with a patient only five minutes a day, in whatever setting, you will not know much about him. It is not possible to decide in advance how much time with a patient is "enough" time for communication to be effective. Some patients may barrage you with words in a five-minute period (and say little); others may virtually say nothing. This is the old problem of individual differences, which must be considered in any facet of nursing care.

Another equally important factor that influences communication with patients is the nurse's ability to communicate verbally, as well as her ability to comprehend nonverbal signs. Nurses too have individual differences. Some have learned to communicate effectively long before they entered nursing; others have yet to learn to do so. Despite these factors, it is still possible to communicate effectively even in a relatively short period of time, and it is possible to learn to do so more skillfully.

The following criteria for studying both your own and the patient's communication may assist you in your efforts to improve your communication. Each of these will be discussed separately.

1. Language
2. Patterns of Verbal and Nonverbal Communication
3. Nurses' Feelings
4. Cultural and Social Factors
5. Stress and Strengths

LANGUAGE

Although language has been discussed earlier, it is necessary to examine several specific aspects of language that either impede or facilitate nurses' communications with patients.

Nurses request patients to do many things, but they frequently do not seem to know how to make requests. In essence, they demand; they do not request. Many requests are made without any rationale given to the patient. The following are examples: "Turn over," "Here, sit up and drink this," "Lie quietly," "Don't move your arm," "Don't cry," "Don't eat your breakfast," *ad infinitum.* One can readily see that these are commands which many people will react to adversely. In addition, they do not provide the patient with any knowledge about their meaning to him as a person.

On the other hand, nurses are quick to react if a patient says, "Bring me a drink of water," "Bring my medicine," or "Call my wife." Nurses frequently respond to these demands with, "You could at least say, please," or as one nurse said, "If that's the way you're going to ask for it, you may have to wait." It's amazing that when the "shoe fits the other foot," it hurts. Obviously, not all nurses demand, or respond to patients' demands in this manner. Many of us do not function very effectively, however, in making requests, and we make our own task more complicated when we demand rather than request with explanation.

Another problem related specifically to language involves trying to find the words to best describe what we mean. We in nursing use many technical words which are foreign to patients. Let us consider the nurse who dashes into a patient's room and announces, "The doctor wants you to have a proctoscopy this a.m.," and then hurries out. The patient will have no idea whether this is a test, a treatment, or a kind of medication. We know the meaning of these words, but patients do not. Some people say, "It's better not to tell the patient, then they won't worry." The problem is that they do worry, even when they are not told. The human being can usually deal with stress if he has an opportunity to organize his resources. The theory of homeostasis confirms this concept.

Patients do not always know the exact words to express how they feel or how to describe their discomforts. Life would be easier for the nurse if the patient could identify "a sharp, stabbing pain, located in my left occipital lobe, or my right lower quadrant." Obviously, they are unable to do this. Because they use words that are not this explicit, we often misunderstand them. A patient may say, "Nurse, I have a lot of pressure." When asked to locate the pressure, the patient responds, "Down here" and points. This is not even a complete sentence, and the words do not tell us very much. In a situation like this, it is necessary to get the patient to explain more precisely what the pressure is like, how it is different from pain, and its exact location. The patient could be describing pressure in the bladder, pressure on the back or buttocks, or at any other area located "down here."

Other examples of this are, "Nurse, I feel sick," or "Nurse, I feel tense," or "Nurse, I'm frightened." These are very general statements which literally have no meaning for action until you have clarified what feeling sick, tense, or frightened means to that person. It is the nurse's responsibility to help the patient verbally describe these feelings. We should never falsely reassure the person with, "Oh, you'll be all right," or "You've nothing to be tense or frightened about."

One patient who told the nurse she "felt sick," was reassured by the nurse that she was o.k. Ten minutes later she vomited a pint of blood. She did not say, "I am nauseated," or even "sick-to-my-stomach." To her, the words "I feel sick" meant nauseated. We must learn to listen to the words, and wonder, "What does he mean by that," and then proceed to have the patient explain further if we are not sure of what he means.

PATTERNS OF VERBAL AND NONVERBAL COMMUNICATION

In a period of over ten years, the examination of nurses' interaction notes revealed that within two or three days patterns of communication appeared between the nurse and the patient. That is, certain topics appeared repeatedly, specific persons were frequently referred to, or particular words or feelings were reiterated. With some patients a specific attitude predominates, and is reflected in the patient's tone of voice.

Each of us uses certain imprecise words or phrases to describe a variety of things. Some people say, "See here," "It's gorgeous," "Darling," or "Sorry about that." But this is somewhat different than patterns of speech which involve the recurrence of a subject throughout various conversations. One recurring theme in this book has been the need for the nurse to listen to the patient's perceptions. It may not have been made explicit, but the underlying topic has been—*listen*. Many times patients are worried about finances, death, their children, etc., and these subjects reappear in their conversations. We should be attuned to these, and at least inquire if this is a particular worry, indicating that you have noticed that the patient mentioned it several times. In this way, you may be able to alleviate a worry if it does exist.

Patterns of communication occur in group meetings. One member tends to generalize, another always wants specific facts or statistics, and yet another clarifies, or summarizes. Some people attempt to verbally deal with feelings being expressed. I do not intend to place a value judgment on these expressions, but only wish to indicate that all of us have patterns of communication, some of which are highly useful.

Nonverbal behaviors likewise occur in patterns. Some people always frown when they are displeased, though they do not verbalize their displeasure. Others pout, bang the nearest available object, or withdraw from the conversation. We can be more helpful to patients if we are alert to, and listen for these patterns.

NURSES' FEELINGS

In any nurse-patient interaction, we have feelings about the patient. We may like a patient because he is polite or because he is considerate of us. We may find him fascinating, jovial, or we may be attracted to him for numerous other reasons. These kinds of feelings rarely interfere with our communication with him. In fact, we may spend more time with him and enjoy caring for him because of them.

We may find other patients annoying, frustrating, sometimes frightening, and generally unlikeable. We find some patients hard to please, demanding of our time, and sometimes so reticent that we don't know what they think. These are the patients that we tend to avoid, to spend little time with, and speak to rather sharply, or not at all. But these people often need our care more than the enjoyable ones.

Our personal feelings about patients are a major influencing factor in our ability to communicate effectively. As such, they may require more effort and attention than any other factor. Each of us reacts to different words, tone of voice, and various behaviors, in our own unique way. What annoys me may not annoy you, and vice versa—our feelings are very personal. There are times when we do not even allow ourselves to be aware of them. This can be extremely troublesome to both parties involved. It is impossible to remedy your feelings if you don't recognize that they exist. Hopefully, some one will help you recognize your feelings toward the patient in order for you to examine what produced these feelings. Usually, this recognition can assist you in reexamining your interaction with the patient and help you resolve your feelings. We must learn to question our reactions and ask ourselves, "What is my feeling toward this patient, and does it interfere in my communication with him?"

In any interaction which produces negative feelings you will need to talk to yourself, identify what produced your feelings, and decide how to resolve them. Suppose that you have a patient who calls you back immediately after you have been in to help him. Clearly, this is extremely annoying, but when it happens, you must realize that you have not helped him, and that you may not know what it is he needs. It is possible to approach him with the attitude that you must not have helped him, because he called you again as soon as you had left the room. If you have this attitude you will have at least given him the benefit of the doubt. Such an attitude will indicate that you are concerned about him. If you really want to help him, your tone of voice will not carry an annoyed quality. More often than not—the patient will tell you his heretofore unexpressed need.

We cannot avoid having negative feelings—nurses are human, but we have a responsibility to do something about them. It is not difficult— we only need to learn how. We must try not to conceal from ourselves the fact that we often fail to react to patients' communication, and deal with *our* own feelings to the neglect of the patient. We must take the initiative; it is a requirement of our role. We, who provide a service to others, carry this responsibility. Most nurses are not indifferent, nor are they unconcerned. Most of us react to feelings stimulated in us by patients' verbal behavior. It would, of course, be worse if we were indifferent and didn't really care. The problem seems to be that we don't know how to deal verbally with persons that produce untoward feelings in us.

CULTURAL AND SOCIAL FACTORS

We in nursing have only begun to take into account the knowledge of cultural and social aspects of health and illness. We have not yet grasped the idea that communication and culture are inseparable.

For clarification, we should make the distinction between culture and society. Dr. Benjamin Paul, a social anthropologist, says they are not identical, but interdependent.

> Among humans, society and culture are interdependent; each can exist only in terms of the other. . . . Where emphasis falls on the ideas shared by a group, the frame of reference is usually cultural. Where emphasis is on the group that shares the ideas, the frame of reference is usually social.[1]

Many of us tend to consider different customs and beliefs as "odd" if they are dissimilar to ours. Edward T. Hall says, in any society the code of manners tends to sum up the culture—to be a frame of reference for all behavior. Our customs regarding cleanliness, manner of eating, how we view time, our differences in attitudes toward space and intimacy all reflect our attitudes and our ability to communicate with each other.[2]

Misunderstandings occur because similar problems arise with patients within our own society. I once knew a very wealthy woman who complained severely about the appearance of her room, the china, and the bed linen, while hospitalized. Staff were angry at her because, "she considered herself better than others." They felt that, "She could jolly well accept what was offered for all patients." They failed to realize that this woman had never before eaten with stainless steel or thick pottery cups, never slept on muslin sheets, nor inhabited a barren room. Her perceptions of her environment repulsed her, and the majority of her conversation centered on these inconveniences of her social world.

From a study done in 1955 by Schatzman and Strauss, it was found that striking differences occurred in communication according to social class. Their data was obtained through interview protocols gathered from participants in a disaster. The participants were defined as middle and lower class with specific criteria describing each class. The difference was "a considerable disparity in (a) the number and kinds of perspectives utilized in communication; (b) the ability to take the listener's role; (c) the handling of classifications; and (d) the frameworks and stylistic devices which order and implement the communication."[3]

Such findings have significance to nursing, as they provide some guidelines for communication with patients of different social classes. Though this is only one study with a relatively small sample of twenty people, it does indicate that members of different social classes see events differently, and thus perceive different meanings. Often we do not take

---

[1]Benjamin D. Paul, *Health, Culture and Community* (New York: Russell Sage Foundation, 1955), pp. 463-464.

[2]Edward T. Hall, "The Anthropology of Manners," *Scientific American*, Vol. 192, No. 4, April, 1955, pp. 84-90.

[3]Leonard Schatzman and A. Strauss, "Social Class and Modes of Communication," A. G. Smith (ed.), *Communication and Culture* (New York: Holt, Rinehart & Winston, Inc., 1966), pp. 442-455.

these differences into consideration. It is these factors that nurses encounter when caring for patients of various ethnic groups.

It is possible that failure to understand a patient's culture will result in a misinterpretation of communication, with consequent harm to the patient. A patient in a psychiatric hospital verbalized what seemed like peculiar ideas about her family. She was seen as psychotic by the staff. The patient was assigned to a student, and an anthropologist was consulted regarding this patient's ethnic group. Through the consultation, it was discovered that the patient's comments were not psychotic—indeed the family was as the patient described. Her communications had led staff to believe that her thinking about her family was distorted!

Anthropologists and various public health officials have conducted a variety of projects in other countries designed to control malaria, teach housewives to boil their drinking water, and instigate various immunization programs. They have found that not all programs are successful because of differences between the perceptions of the populations served and the perceptions of the project staff. What was communicated, how it was communicated, and who communicated, were factors that facilitated or impeded acceptance of the changes.

It has become evident in nursing that the integration of mental health concepts into the basic curriculum has not always been successful. Likewise, public health nurses have been forced to accept patients with mental health problems in their case load. Public health and medical-surgical nurses have been offered consultation, but in some instances they have not utilized the services. If we could study these situations, we would doubtless find that there was a communication breakdown somewhere in the process. Frequently, we have not studied their situations, nor have we ascertained their reception to the idea. If we are to introduce changes to improve health practices, we must learn what the people involved think, regardless of the country.

In examining nurse-patient communication, cultural and social aspects must be considered. Both are factors which alter our communication with each other. Some patients may receive poor nursing care because we do not understand these factors.

STRESS AND STRENGTHS

These two criteria, necessary for examining the patient's communication, will be discussed together. Most persons who are suffering from ill health, physical or psychological (though they are not separate), endure some degree of stress. Of course, not all stress is disabling; in fact, it serves a useful purpose in assisting the individual to harness his resources for positive action. The word *stress* is one of those words that has different meanings for various people. Hans Selye discusses the semantic difficulties he encountered when he first attempted to explain biological stress. After eliminating several words as unsuitable, he retained the word "stress" which he felt best described his concept. The concept of stress is an abstraction, and Selye describes its medical sense as "essentially the rate of wear and tear on the body. Anyone who feels that whatever he is doing—or whatever is being done to him—is strenuous and wearing, knows vaguely what we mean by stress. The feelings of just being tired, jittery, or ill are subjective sensations of stress."[4]

Karl Menninger accepts G. L. Engel's definition of stress as follows:

> Psychological stress refers to all processes, whether originating in the external environment or within the person, which impose a demand or requirement upon the organism the resolution or handling of which requires . . . activity of the mental apparatus before any other system is involved or activated.[5]

Stephen Horsley contends that stress disorder is due primarily to faulty interpersonal relationships, and states. "Three main fields of potential stress are the family, one's work mates, and the community, but none of these can be evaluated in isolation because conflict in any one threatens each of the others."[6] It is appropriate here to point out that "tension" is a synonym for stress, and the words will be used interchangeably.

A great deal more could be written regarding stress, but many authorities would agree with the concepts presented. Our purpose here relates to the recognition that stress exists in any form of illness. It thereby becomes a factor with which the nurse must concern herself in communicating with patients. The first step is to recognize that stress does exist. The degree of stress varies from individual to individual, and the source of stress may be different. For some patients, the stress may be directly related to their illness. For others, the main source may be from the family, the job, or some external factor. The second step is to ascertain the source of the stress, recognizing that at times we may also be a source of stress as well.

After spending some time in a general hospital, the following verbalizations were made by patients indicating sources of stress: "What if I yell or scream during labor?" "I hope I don't say things I shouldn't when

---

4Hans Selye, *The Stress of Life* (New York: McGraw-Hill Book Company, 1956), p. 3.

5Karl Menninger, *The Vital Balance* (New York: The Viking Press, 1963), p. 129.

6Stephen Horsley, "Creative Tension," *Nursing Times*, Vol. 63, June 30, 1967, p. 867.

I wake up from the anesthesia"; "I can't imagine what it feels like to have abdominal surgery"; "They don't seem to know what's wrong with me"; and "Do stitches ever really not hold?" These are questions which cannot be passed off as inconsequential, even if we have heard them a million times. The patient needs reassurance from you about what your reaction will be, or specific information where indicated. The third step involves your responses which will alleviate the stress.

Mary Meyers' study of three approaches to assisting patients indicated that, "Less tension is created when the patient is given specific information upon which he can structure the event of impending stress."[7] In this study, she introduced a new procedure to three groups of patients, with the expectation that the unfamiliarity of the stimulus situation would produce a mild degree of stress. As the new procedure was introduced, each group was given one of three different conditions of communication. Her results showed that: (1) a "structuring" communication—designed to explain the situation to the patient produced less tension; (2) a "no" communication, in which the patient was told nothing produced less tension in the patient than (3) an "irrelevant" communication designed to distract or divert attention from the procedure. In the "structured" communication, the patient felt he was no longer a depersonalized patient being treated in a routine way. Tension was produced by distracting communication, and this approach was the least desirable for tension reduction. Less tension was created when nothing was said, than when what was said was irrelevant.

This example refers to stress from the external environment, instigated by a nursing procedure. When an explanation is made, the person has an opportunity to prepare for the stress and can more adequately cope with it. The unknown, as in this study when no information was given, often is more frightening to individuals. Though some tension was created by providing no information, even more tension was produced by irrelevant information. What reduces stress or tension in various kinds of situations needs much more study than has been done so far. Although this is one of the primary functions of the nurse, we have practically no scientific evidence to give us answers.

We must keep in mind that the human being has an inherent ability to cope with far more stress than we sometimes realize. The fact that some patients have endured thirty years in a mental hospital attests to this fact. If we had recognized the "strengths" these people possessed, we might have helped them recognize and develop these strengths for

[7]Mary Meyers, "The Effects of Communication on Patients' Reactions to Stress," *Nursing Research*, Spring, 1964, p. 131.

coping with their problems. We have focused so long on people's limitations or diseases, that we have overlooked their assets.

Dr. Halbert Dunn says that perhaps disease is more interesting, and "that it's easier to fight *against* sickness than to fight *for* a condition of greater wellness." He uses the term *high level wellness* to mean "an integrated method of functioning which is oriented toward maximizing the potential of which the individual is capable within the environment where he is functioning."[8] Dr. Dunn is not implying that there is an optimum level of wellness, "but rather that wellness is a *direction in progress* toward an even higher potential of functioning."[9] We must help patients recognize their assets; it gives them strength to develop their potentials. Even with the most "complaining" patient, it is more helpful to say, "I think you do remarkably well considering your many problems," than it is to say, "Do you always complain so much?" The former statement indicates that the patient has strength to cope with the many problems; in the latter you indicate a weakness. Sometimes it is necessary to remind a patient who is chastizing himself, "Look at yourself, you have your strong points, so don't discount them."

Herbert Otto, Chairman of the Human Potentialities Research Project at the University of Utah, supports this view. In eighteen experimental groups of healthy or "normal" people of all ages, and in diverse professions, he found they had a clearer concept of their problems or weaknesses than of their strengths or assets. He speaks specifically to nurses when he says that the "Nurse's major contribution to the patient lies in what she communicates to him attitudinally, what she conveys to him about himself, his outlook, and his prospects for the future." He further states: "The fact that the average person functions at only ten to fifteen per cent of his potential presents a major challenge."[10] The nurse who can communicate the awareness of the potential which she possesses as a part of her professional function instills hope and encourages the development of health processes, while at the same time helping her to clarify her professional use of herself. May I remind you that his concept is useful to all people—not just patients.

Erik Erikson describes inherent strengths of humans as virtues, which are human qualities of strength, related to that process by which ego strength may be developed and imparted from generation to generation. Hope, Will, Purpose, and Competence are rudiments of virtue in childhood. Fidelity is the virtue of adolescence, and Love, Care, and Wisdom

---

[8]Halbert Dunn, *High Level Wellness* (Washington, D. C.: Mount Vernon Publishing Company, Inc., 1961), pp. 3-4.

[9]*Ibid.*, p. 6.

[10]Herbert Otto, "The Human Potentialities of Nurses and Patients," *Nursing Outlook*, August, 1965, pp. 32-35.

occur as virtues in adulthood.[11] The latter three are certainly strengths that nurses need to possess to fulfill their functions adequately.

Verbal and nonverbal interactions with patients can be examined, using the five criteria discussed: (1) Language, the words we use and the tone of voice accompanying the words; (2) the various patterns of both verbal and nonverbal communication; (3) the cultural and social forces that impinge on our expressions; (4) nurse's feelings about individual patients; and (5) identifying the kind of stress the patient is experiencing as well as identifying with the patient the strengths he uses to cope with his stresses.

Nurses' communication and that of patients should be examined by these criteria. If we would utilize this framework for reviewing our communication, we could become skillful, and would have a comprehensive profile of satisfactory and unsatisfactory communication areas of both nurses and patients.

BIBLIOGRAPHY

DUNN, HALBERT. *High Level Wellness*. Washington, D. C.: Mount Vernon Publishing Company, Inc., 1961.

ERIKSON, ERIK H. *Insight and Responsibility*. New York: W. W. Norton & Company, Inc., 1964.

HALL, EDWARD T. "The Anthropology of Manners," *Scientific American*, Vol. 192, No. 4, April, 1955.

HORSLEY, STEPHEN. "Creative Tension." *Nursing Times*, June 30, 1967.

MENNINGER, KARL A. *The Vital Balance*. New York: The Viking Press, 1963.

MEYERS, MARY. "The Effects of Communication on Patients' Reaction to Stress," *Nursing Research*, Spring, 1964.

OTTO, HERBERT. "The Human Potentialities of Nurses and Patients," *Nursing Outlook*, August, 1965.

PAUL, BENJAMIN, D. *Health, Culture and Community*. New York: Russell Sage Foundation, 1955.

SCHATZMAN, LEONARD, and STRAUSS, A. "Social Class and Modes of Communication," A. G. Smith (ed.), *Communication and Culture*. New York: Holt, Rinehart & Winston, Inc., 1966.

SELYE, HANS. *The Stress of Life*. New York: McGraw-Hill Book Company, 1956.

---

[11]Erik H. Erikson, *Insight and Responsibility* (New York: W. W. Norton & Company, Inc., 1964), pp. 111-157.

Imaginative Nurses

The gratification that one experiences from successful communication with another person can be an ideal of individual fulfillment. Each of us strives for meaning with his fellowman. Along with this is the need to strive for excellence. The pursuit of excellence is best described by John W. Gardner in the following remarks:

> Keeping a free society free—and vital and strong—is no job for the half-educated and the slovenly. Free men must be competent. . . . But excellence implies more than competence. It implies a striving for the highest standards in every phase of life. We need individual excellence in all its forms—in every kind of creative endeavor, in political life, in education, in industry—in short, universally.[1]

This also applies to nursing. It is not easy to strive for excellence, but can we really afford to settle for less? Questions constantly arise in life which demand answers. Patients need imaginative nurses. We need to develop intellectual curiosity, rather than to settle for "intellectual anemia." We in nursing have moved from a "procedure oriented type of action" to a "thinking behavior." We can no longer rely on stereotyped opinions and beliefs. We must begin to think creatively, which requires such alternatives as, "What should I have done differently?" or "What should I have said differently?"

CREATIVE THINKING

Creative thinking is a major factor in the accomplishment of our tasks. Thinking critically or creatively are concepts we use which often have

---

[1]John W. Gardner, *Excellence* (New York: Harper & Row, Publishers, 1961), pp. 159-160.

little meaning for us. We use them frequently, but what things came to mind when you read the sentence, "Creative thinking is a main factor in the accomplishment of our tasks"? The statement infers a commitment to something (creative thinking), and a commitment to accomplish our tasks (nursing). We in nursing are pledged to both; the latter is specifically included in our code of ethics, and in present day society we cannot accomplish the latter without the former.

How does one think creatively? Is it different than ordinary thinking? Is it different than critical thinking? Any time you recognize that a relationship exists between an observation about a patient's care or condition that you have not been aware of previously is a creative thought. William H. Burton, *et al.*, say it more elaborately, "The production of insights which cut through confusion to reach the heart of the matter, the sudden flash of so-called inspiration, or intuition are all creative processes." A second kind of creative thinking, as stated by the same authors, is the production of something "new, unique, not-before-existent."[2] If, through your originality, you discovered a new approach for establishing patients' trust in you, or discovered a new way of determining the number of respirations per minute, or developed a teaching program for young mothers in the ghetto, you would be utilizing a process of creative thinking.

We have assumed for so long that the way we do things now is the correct way, and these assumptions frequently impede our progress. Nurses have assumed for years that the majority of patients automatically trust them. Some studies indicate that this is a false assumption. Hanging on to false assumptions is an obstacle to progress. Similarly, in our communication with one another, we frequently assume that the patient knows what we are talking about. To be creative requires that you examine current assumptions on which any problem rests and reason them through to determine if they are accurate.

FACTS VERSUS OPINIONS

In conjunction with assumptions, one hears a great deal of talk about "getting the facts." Why do we get facts? How do we mean something? We gather facts to solve problems, and from the inferences we can make from these facts, we gain knowledge based on our final interpretation of the facts. Sometimes we become defensive when we have stated "a fact" and someone says, "Are you certain that is a fact?" If you said, "You can't talk to that patient, he absolutely refuses to listen," is this

---

[2]Wm. H. Burton, R. B. Kimball, and R. L. Wing, *Education for Effective Thinking* (New York: Appleton-Century-Crofts, 1960), p. 324.

a fact? One would need to examine whether this statement is based on one or more interactions, whether it was verified by others, what had been said by the nurse, and what kind of subject was discussed. How can I possibly know if this is an accurate statement about the patient, unless I proceed by "gathering other facts"?

Many times, particularly if we have a discussion on something we feel strongly about, we generalize from a single incident. We arrive at a belief which is not a fact. Wm. H. Burton, *et al.*, discuss the ways in which we obtain facts: (1) observation through our senses, (2) observations through instruments of precision, (3) an experimental procedure, (4) use of printed sources, and (5) other persons.* When information is received from a single source, it is often necessary for us to double-check it so that we can be sure it is fact and not merely an opinion. This does not necessarily mean that the source is incompetent but that certain information was lacking about the interaction which precluded acceptance of the conclusion offered.

COMMUNICATING OUR OBSERVATIONS

In nursing we rely on our observations for enormous amounts of information about patients. Many of our observations are faulty. One good reason for this is that we always observe from our own frame of reference. This is why cameras are used at Olympic games; it is easier to see the U.S. runner in front, because of our frame of reference. The camera removes this bias—it is one of the precision instruments. During an emergency, who did what, and when, varies to a degree with every person observing.

Each of us reacts to, or looks for a specific occurrence, and ignores certain other specifics. This could be one advantage of having several nurses work with one patient. Each could observe the patient, and "see" him differently. Each nurse could communicate in her own manner, and gain additional knowledge about the patient. This presumes that one nurse would not be unduly influenced by the other and could make her own inferences.

We need evidence on which to base our actions, and it must be accurate evidence. For example, a particular nurse described a patient in the following manner: "I haven't really talked to her, but I have watched her. She seemed so dominating and superficial, that I walked away from her." These sensory observations led to a belief about this person, which in turn led to an avoidance of her. Since the nurse made no attempt to

---

*For a detailed description of each, see Chapter 6, pp. 74-109.

verbally validate her observations, she was acting solely on opinion. How the nurse would have verbally dealt with her observations cannot be known, but if she believed her observations were correct, her verbalizations would not have assisted the patient.

This nurse's observations of the patient also influenced her attitude or belief, and caused the nurse's comments about the patient to be derogatory. She did not have an open-mind of inquiry. Her values about a kind of behavior interfered with her role as a helping person. The evidence for her actions was incomplete. The situations called for critical thinking, which requires a suspension of judgment until further inquiry is made. Other interpretations could have been made of the behavior observed. All of these factors (the sensory observations, the nurse's attitude, the nurse's values, and the nurse's thinking) may seem unrelated, but they show one important element. They all depend on communication. What the nurse communicated about the patient was a result of these factors.

We, as nurses, must become cognizant that we are often more "self-centered" than "other person centered," as revealed in the above example. Furthermore, our standards of behavior may not be the same as the patient's standards. It is not a matter of right or wrong standards, but a matter of recognizing differences and learning how to mediate them. We have the responsibility for taking the initiative in communicating with the patient. We cannot jump to conclusions, based on our own expectations.

It can be very gratifying to assist patients in making their own decisions. By exploring with the patient, it is possible to assist him in anticipating various consequences resulting from alternative decisions. A young student nurse once illustrated this while working with a teen-age girl. The patient was annoyed that she could not smoke on the elevator, stating, "There are rules wherever you go, and I am not going to pay any attention." The student asked what she thought would occur if she lit a cigarette. "I'll be told to put it out." The student then asked if she preferred to do as she wished and risk being embarrassed. The patient refrained and said, "I suppose the rule is made because the elevator is so crowded; it would be easy to burn someone." The nurse agreed. It is always more profitable to allow the other person to examine the situation and make his own decisions based on reasoning and anticipating consequences, than to deny him this experience. Nurses must allow patients the time to incorporate new ideas, and assist them in examining alternatives to arrive at more logical reasoning.

It is not easy to learn to communicate effectively, but the rewards are very gratifying if we attempt to do so. Most of us fail to recognize that we have deficiencies in this area. Thus, the first step is to examine our communication and look for our deficiencies, and then to proceed to develop our skills. We must learn to demand much of ourselves if we wish to successfully carry out our role as a helping person in society. I hope no one has led you to believe that this role is an easy one. It isn't; it requires the maximum use of your potentials.

RECORDING

A few comments are necessary regarding nurses' recordings related to patient care. It can be estimated that within the near future the mass of the data we have customarily recorded will be processed by computer. Medications, vital signs, and various laboratory reports will be recorded automatically. Doubtless we will develop means of recording behavioral manifestations as well. Our function will be to provide the necessary descriptions of human behavior that will give an accurate picture of the patient. Perhaps we can devise a system that will enable us to identify patients' needs more accurately, based on the descriptions we provide the computer. The main purpose of any recording is to provide information to all disciplines involved in the care of the patient in order to restore the patient to a maximum state of health. Otherwise we have no need for the information. It is a challenge to seek means of recording information that benefits the patient.

SUMMARY

Throughout the book an attempt has been made to convey the importance of communication in all our interactions with others, but particularly in nurses' interactions with patients. Various aspects of verbal and nonverbal communication have been examined in order to help you gain an appreciation of the value of successful communication. We can no longer ignore this responsibility in our work with patients. You cannot care for patients adequately and be unaware of this dimension of nursing. Communication is an integral part of all nursing, and has not received sufficient emphasis in the past. Some nurses have been aware of this necessity in psychiatric nursing, but it is also necessary for the nurse caring for medical, surgical, pediatric, and other in-patients as well as the patient in the home or in the community.

I hope that the basic information provided here will help you to become more cognizant of your communication and the communication of your patients. You should make it an active concern of your daily endeavors. Though this is only an introduction to the field of communication, it is presented with the hope that it will whet your appetite for further investigation. The benefits will be gratifying and challenging. It is through communication that you have the opportunity to show concern, understanding, and compassion to your patients. I hope you accept the challenge.

BIBLIOGRAPHY

BURTON, WM. H. R.; KIMBALL, R. B.; and WING, R. E. *Education for Effective Thinking*. New York: Appleton-Century-Crofts, 1960.
GARDNER, JOHN W. *Excellence*. New York: Harper & Row, Publishers, 1961.

Index

105